be good
to your gut

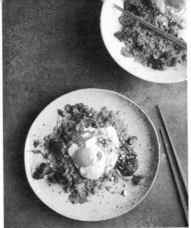

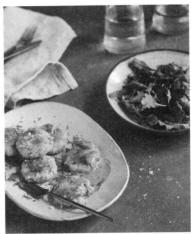

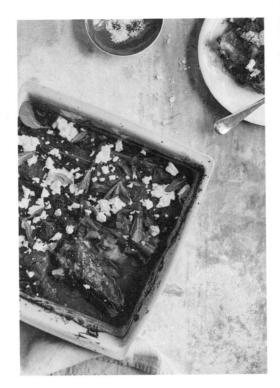

be good
to your gut

The ultimate guide to gut health –
with 80 delicious recipes to feed
your body and mind

eve kalinik

piatkus

PIATKUS

First published in Great Britain in 2017 by Piatkus
Copyright © Eve Kalinik 2017

A CIP catalogue record for this book is available from the British Library.

ISBN: 978-0-349-41492-8

All photography © Nassima Rothacker
Food stylist: Rosie Ramsden
Book design: D.R. ink
Editors: Maggie Ramsay and Jillian Stewart
Printed and bound in Germany Mohn Media

Papers used by Piatkus are from well-managed forests and other responsible sources.

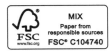

MIX
Paper from
responsible sources
FSC® C104740

Piatkus
An imprint of Little, Brown Book Group, Carmelite House, 50 Victoria Embankment, London EC4Y 0DZ

An Hachette UK Company
www.hachette.co.uk

www.improvementzone.co.uk

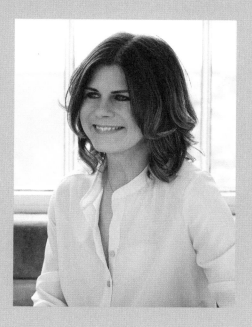

Eve Kalinik BA Hons, Dip NT, mBANT, CNHC, is regarded as one of the most exciting voices in food and health today. Her modern, fresh and innovative approach to gut health, which combines scientific knowledge and practical advice with inspiring and delicious recipes, means she is in great demand as a nutritional therapist, and as a columnist and consultant. Aside from her nutritional practice, Eve is a columnist for *Psychologies* and matchesfashion.com, a frequent speaker at various industry events and one of the tutors for *Guardian* Masterclasses.

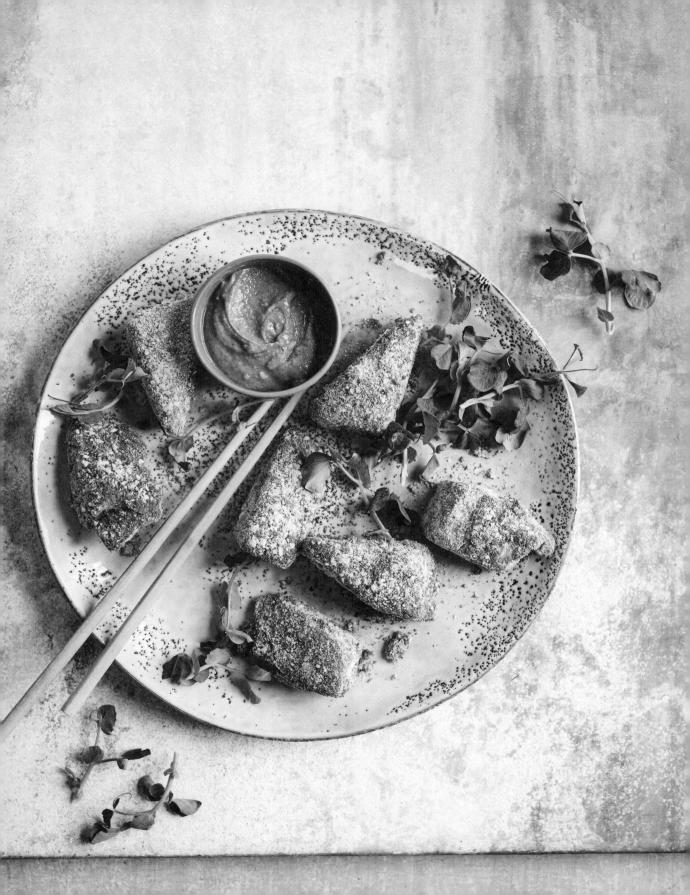

contents

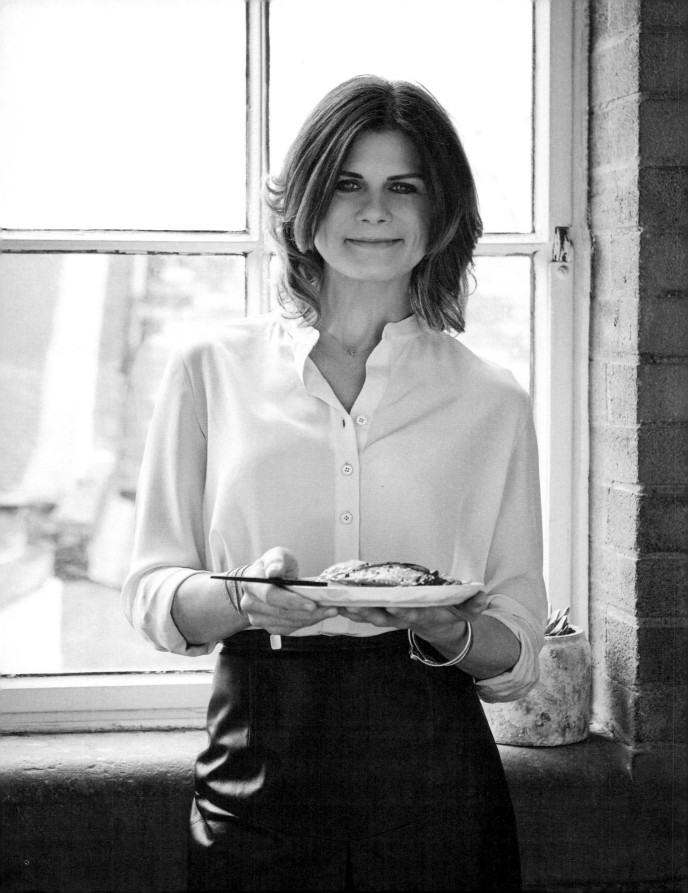

introduction

OK, SO I CONFESS, I'm a bit of a mad-keen foodie. I genuinely don't think there is anything more fulfilling than enjoying a plate of good, honest, delicious food with great company and usually a decent drop of natural red on the side. I'm passionate about how eating well can make such a big difference to our health and wellbeing. And as a nutritional therapist who has a particular interest in gut health, I love sharing my enthusiasm for all things tasty and how food affects us from the inside out. However, my passion for food wasn't always so geared towards the more wholesome options. Before learning about what good food really means, I was often a slave to some of the boxed, bagged and convenience 'ding-when-it's-done' stuff.

Indeed I grew up as part of the generation whose diet was somewhat lacking in natural foods and was instead generously peppered with garish-coloured concoctions, packet desserts and artificial ingredients. I remember being mesmerised by the likes of blue icy beverages or skipping to the local shop for a treat of pick 'n' mix sweets. Of course, many of us were none the wiser about the long-term impact that a lack of fresh produce and regular consumption of nutritionally devoid and chemically enhanced foods could have on the trillions of microbes that reside in the gut – and on our health in general.

I think it's fair to say that, all things considered, we stamped an altogether abysmal mark on the health of our gut. And yet, despite greater

The real work on getting your gut to the best place possible naturally starts with what you feed it. And no, you don't need to buy expensive powders and supplements or follow some unsustainable regime.

awareness of the vital role that eating well plays in good health, many people still find themselves woefully disassociated from the food on the plate in front of them. I put a lot of blame for this disconnection on the rapidly changing face of modern life, which has particular ramifications for the gut. One of these changes is our over-zealous habit of pill popping. Gone are the days of our grandmother's natural remedies – if there's a pill for it, we take it. For anyone who has their head buried in the sand on this one, it's widely recognised that things like excessive use of painkillers can really mess with the gut. And, as if that isn't enough for our poor beleaguered digestive systems to handle, we are also under more stress than ever. Greater work and financial responsibilities – and the ridiculously long working hours inherent in our 24/7 online world – leave us practically zero time to 'rest and digest'.

Given all these pressures, is it really any wonder that digestive problems are ubiquitous and that the number of sufferers seems to be rising? The fact that symptoms such as bloating, gas and even debilitating pain are seen as 'normal' is just plain wrong. It seems that many of us have become so far removed from listening and tuning into our gut that we simply choose to look the other way and ignore it. Or we might be coming up against a brick wall time and time again and are unable to find answers or clues to symptoms that may have been going on for years.

my story

My story is not an unusual one and indeed it might sound familiar to a lot of you. I was actually a pretty robust child. That might have had something to do with having a father of Polish descent who was forever fermenting things (his *bigos* – sauerkraut and meat stew – is still the best you will ever taste). My mother was also a proficient pickler, who invariably cooked everything from scratch and in the most traditional way possible. So despite being a typical teenager and having the odd junk food blowout now and then, I had a fairly balanced diet that gave my gut an excellent grounding. Things took a turn for the worse, however, following a trip abroad, where I picked up a pretty nasty parasite. What followed were years of digestive symptoms that I just kind of 'managed'. Some days were good but most were bad.

At the end of my time at university I started to suffer from recurrent kidney infections that resulted in prescription after prescription for antibiotics. At one point I was taking them on a daily basis prophylactically to prevent yet another infection. To say my gut was unhappy doesn't begin to describe the miserable state I was in. I was constantly bloated, constipated and often in a lot of pain, but with no other option than to dutifully swallow my daily dose of antibiotics. Little did I know that in attempting to wipe out the kidney infections

I was haphazardly killing all the bacteria in my gut – including the beneficial ones. Moreover, this left my gut like an open playing field for more pathogenic species to grow and, unbeknown to me, slowly destroy my immune system. The more antibiotics I took, the worse it got. At the time, I had a full-on career in fashion. I was at the top of my game – or should have been – but dealing with the pressures of a high-profile job while trying desperately to manage my symptoms left me near breaking point. In short, my gut was a mess – and so was I.

The fact that symptoms such as bloating, gas and even debilitating pain are seen as 'normal' is just plain wrong.

I knew deep down that how I was feeling wasn't right. There had to be a solution. So, taking what little knowledge I had at the time and with a huge amount of determination, I set out on a mission to find it. Countless medical, holistic and off-the-wall specialists later (and a whole lot poorer to boot), I ended up back where I'd begun with the same symptoms. It was soul destroying.

It was at this low point that I started reading more about nutrition, food and, most importantly, the gut. And something quite magical began to happen. With small changes to my diet, my digestive symptoms improved, and little by little I weaned myself off antibiotics. The changes were small but had a profound effect. I was shocked at just how important a role food had to play in my health. Feeling empowered but still a long

way from where I wanted to be, I went to see a nutritionist who, after running some tests, confirmed that my gut had indeed suffered a battering and my gut bacteria were totally out of balance and dominated by some pretty nasty microbes. It was time to take real action. Armed with tailored guidance on my diet, I began eating fermented, probiotic and gut-supportive foods, some of which I had previously considered 'unhealthy', such as unpasteurised full fat cheese. Just as importantly, I began removing some seemingly 'healthy' foods that I thought had been helping, such as low calorie cereals.

With the addition of a couple of targeted supplements, I managed to regain my health and, crucially, that of my gut. The problems I'd suffered over the years had started there after all and giving my gut the support that it so desperately needed got me back on track. It may sound a little clichéd but food really had become my medicine. Fast forward a few more months that were packed with relentless travelling and stressful events and I was beginning to feel that it was time to hang up my hat in the fashion game. Inspired by how my own health had been dramatically transformed, I decided that I wanted to help people improve their health in the same way, so I began training to be a nutritional therapist.

understanding your inside story

Nutritional therapy, for those of you who are not familiar with it, means using food and natural supplementation to bring the body into homeostasis, or balance. For me, that fundamentally starts with the gut. My personal journey aside, I have not met one person in my clinic, workshops or events who can honestly say they have perfect digestion. I genuinely don't think it exists in this day and age. The good news is that by working with our inner ecosystem, and tending it as we would a garden, we can get one that is pretty damn close to perfect. Indeed, the gut is one of the most fascinating ecosystems you could ever imagine, with its very own rolling landscapes, rich soil and diversity of species. Unsurprisingly, as more is uncovered about its central role in health, the gut has become a massive area of research in recent years.

We are only beginning to gain some understanding of the true complexity of the gut and why it is of such paramount importance in our overall health. That vital, underpinning role kind of makes sense really, given that there are more bacteria than human cells in the body. Recent figures put it at a 1.5:1 ratio, and when you consider that most of these bacteria reside in the gut it provides more than a little food for thought. That fact alone should inspire you to get more up close and personal with your gut. And that's why I wrote this book: to help you reconnect with your gut and all that it can do for your health, and to empower you to be able to make the necessary changes, as I once did.

how this book can help you

The real work on getting your gut to the best place possible naturally starts with what you feed it. And no, you don't need to buy expensive powders and supplements or follow some unsustainable regime. It's all about understanding and nourishing your body with the foods that really count. These are the ones that will truly nourish your gut and allow all those trillions of microbes to flourish. Throughout the book I'll be guiding you through the foods that will best support your gut and, of course, providing lots of delicious, digestion-friendly recipes. I'll also be encouraging you to reintroduce some foods that you probably thought you needed to banish for good. Foods such as cheese, milk and bread, made the traditional way, can all support you on the way to a blissfully happy gut. And I hope to inspire you to become a fellow fermenter by demonstrating how easy it is to make foods like sauerkraut and kefir, which you can have every day and that give so much back to your gut. I'll also explain why nothing can take the place of an enriched and plentiful diet, and look at the many pitfalls and saboteurs that can stand in your way. There are a lot of strange concepts out there concerning nutrition — and a lot of confusion — so I'll help demystify a lot of that, too.

I hope this book will give you a deeper and more practical understanding of why having a strong and healthy gut doesn't simply improve digestion — it has a profound effect on almost every aspect of our health and wellbeing. Some of the information will really surprise you, but I think most of it will inspire you and help you to take your health into your own hands.

Each chapter deals with the significant role that the gut has to play in areas such as our mental health, immune system, hormones and stress. It doesn't matter who you are, how you live, your age … everyone has something to gain from learning how to support their gut. Whether you simply want to optimise your health, address certain areas of personal concern or make sense of some of the issues that may have been affecting you for years, I want to help you tread that path a little more smoothly and with the honest facts to hand.

One thing is for sure, this isn't a diet book. There is nothing extreme or quick fix here. This book is designed to give you the know-how to make long-term changes, so there are no punishing regimes that will cause you to fall at the first hurdle. It is about balance and having a healthy mindset, so by all means indulge in the odd glass of good quality wine or piece of freshly baked cake when you fancy it. Having a healthy gut isn't about being saintly with your choices all the time but about becoming more informed and basing

It is about understanding and nourishing your body with the foods that really count. These are the ones that will truly nourish your gut and allow all those trillions of microbes to flourish.

your diet on foods that nourish you. Even if you start with one simple thing, that's a huge achievement, and a big step forwards in the health of your gut. So come back to this book time and time again, trying different recipes and foods and incorporating healthier habits into your routine gradually and consistently. That's what will have the most significant impact, after all.

You'll be relieved to hear that you don't need to have a Michelin star or be a whizz kid in the kitchen to follow my recipes. They are simple to make, lip-smackingly good and, best of all, brilliant for your gut. The recipes complement the subject of each chapter and will help you to put all of the knowledge you gain throughout

the book into practice. They'll also prove wholeheartedly that healthy, great tasting food isn't an oxymoron.

Making your own meals from scratch will soon become second nature and will help you rediscover a sense of respect and appreciation for food, which is so important for good gut health and the process of digestion. We can all benefit from having a better emotional relationship with our food and for me that fundamentally means eating at a table with real gratitude, joy and our taste buds firing.

With the knowledge on how to help rebalance and support the gut, and a newfound spark of inspiration in the kitchen, you can begin to make real, lasting changes. When it comes to the gut, I like to use the analogy of a garden: you need the right soil for the flowers to bloom and regular weeding to enable them to thrive. Think of it as weeding out hindering factors, such as pests, and using the right nutrients and the proverbial watering can to encourage the good stuff to flourish. Tend your gut well, give it the care and attention it truly deserves and you can build a strong, happy and lifelong partnership.

With that in mind, let's start this journey together, sitting and eating our food with anticipation and glee and giving a hearty toast to the gut and its many microbes – you are wonderful!

On the following pages you'll find some guidance on the most important staple ingredients that I use in the recipes. Please read this before getting those creative juices flowing in the kitchen.

my must-have basic ingredients

As far as possible, ingredients should be organic or from local farmers' markets. In particular eggs, meat and poultry should be non-negotiably organic, free range or grass fed. Dairy milk should be organic, full fat unhomogenised or raw, and cheese unpasteurised. You can read more about unpasteurised dairy foods in Chapter 6, and more about choosing organic in Chapter 10.

milk – you should always opt for full fat, organic and unhomogenised dairy milk. As this is closest to its natural state, it is easier on digestion and provides all the benefits of the fat-soluble vitamins. Raw (unpasteurised) milk is my preferred choice as you reap all of the probiotic and digestive enzyme benefits. See my shopping guide (page 264) on where to source raw milk. If you are vegan, have a go at making your own plant-based milks (see Chapter 6); if you are buying vegan milk, ensure that you go for the unsweetened versions.

water – I recommend always using filtered water when preparing recipes. This is because clean pure water is a crucial part of good nutrition and filtering removes many of the substances that can be present in tap water. You can use natural mineral water if it is in glass bottles, but avoid plastic bottles as these may contain unwanted chemicals and they

I often use ingredients that you won't find in the average cookbook. Don't panic! Turn to my shopping guide on page 260 to find out more about these.

suck for the environment, too. Investing in a good filtration system is better for your health and more cost effective in the long run. Have a look at my shopping guide (page 266) for a recommended filtration system. Water is also discussed in Chapter 10.

oils – When choosing oils, always go for organic, cold pressed versions and extra virgin when it comes to olive oil. Cold pressed means that no heat is used in the extraction process and so the oils retain more of their nutritional value and flavour. They are also not subject to oxidisation from light or heat, which can change their chemical structure. This is why a good rule of thumb is to invest in good quality oils that are sold in dark glass bottles to protect them from the light. The cheap vegetable-based cooking oils in clear plastic bottles won't be cold pressed, so avoid these like the plague. But as with any unrefined cold pressed oils, as a general rule of thumb, use them for drizzling instead of cooking at high temperatures. You can use pure olive oil, which is different to extra virgin. However, heating many of these unrefined cold pressed oils can alter their chemical structure, which diminishes their nutrition and flavour benefits.

The oils that are generally better for cooking at high heat are the ones that are solid at room temperature; these healthy saturated fats have a high smoke point so can be used for cooking at high temperatures. I often use coconut oil, which has natural anti-fungal, anti-microbial and anti-parasitic properties. They are also excellent for keeping the microbiome – the body's bacterial population, the majority of which is found in the gut – in good order.

Other healthy saturated fats include organic unsalted butter (ideally raw or cultured), ghee (clarified butter, meaning most of the milk proteins have been removed) or pork lard from pasture-raised animal. These pastured animal fats provide a wealth of nutritional benefits. Read more about butter in Chapter 9.

mineral-rich salt

mineral-rich salt – Buying salt that is unrefined and rich with minerals, such as natural sea salt, rather than the free-flowing table salt that has been stripped of all its nutritional value, is really important. Read more about salt in Chapter 8. You can find unrefined salt in most supermarkets; look for brands such as Maldon or Halen Môn.

sweetening

sweetening – I have chosen not to use refined sugar in the book as we all know excessive consumption is not great for your health. Read more on this in Chapter 7.

My preferred sweetener is raw honey as it contains bountiful amounts of enzymes and antioxidants that give our gut microbial army a boost (read about this in Chapter 4). However, it is important to get raw honey and not the processed, heat-treated and filtered honey you find in most food shops; this processing removes all of the nutritional benefits that you find in the raw stuff. Your local health food store or farm shop is a good place to look.

nut butters

nut butters – Where possible, opt for the organic versions, and definitely those without any added sugar or sweeteners – really you just want nuts and possibly a bit of salt, that's it! You can also buy sprouted and activated versions of cashew and almond butter, which are even more nutritious and gut friendly. Have a look at my shopping guide for some recommended brands.

storage and cooking

When storing your food opt for glass and ceramic containers over plastic as much as possible for environmental, nutritional and flavour benefits. Some plastic containers potentially harbour chemical substances. Don't worry if that's all you have, but definitely avoid putting piping hot food in them and gradually replace them with ceramic and glass alternatives.

For cooking, invest in pans that are not coated with chemicals – see my kitchen kit list on page 265 for some recommendations.

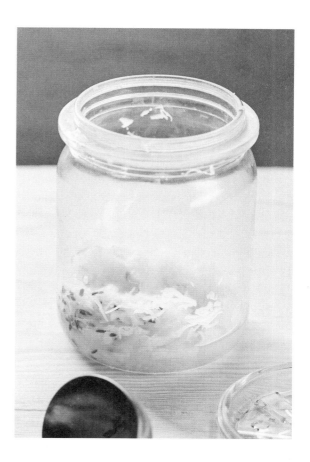

activating nuts and seeds

You will see that many of the recipes call for 'activated' nuts and seeds. This means soaking and drying them, and depending on the nut or seed they will require different soaking times (see chart). Why is this necessary? Well, soaking is important to help remove or reduce 'anti-nutrients' such as phytic acid and other substances that can impair our absorption of nutrients and may also cause irritation to the gut. To learn more about this, see page 98. Soaking also gives a smoother texture when you come to blend nuts and seeds.

To soak, you need to just about cover your nuts or seeds in filtered water with a teaspoon of mineral-rich salt and leave for the time specified in the chart. After that nuts or seeds need to be thoroughly drained and rinsed. If you are not using them immediately for a cream, dressing or something similar they also need to be dried.

To dry them you can either use a dehydrator at 42°C or an oven set to its lowest temperature (usually around 50°C). You will need to dry them for around 12 hours in the dehydrator and 5–10 hours in the oven (depending on how low your oven goes), but check to make sure they are fully dried before you store them away. I would advise that you do a big batch across all your nuts and seeds and store in sealable glass jars ready for use in other recipes or just to eat as a snack. *Voila* – activated nuts and seeds!

You will have to do this prep in advance and although it takes time, it doesn't demand a lot of your attention. And it's worth it.

food	soaking time (hours)
Adzuki beans	8–12
Almonds*	8–12
Amaranth	8
Barley	6
Black beans	8–12
Brazil nuts*	3–4
Buckwheat	6
Butterbeans	7–8
Cashews*	2–4
Chickpeas	8
Flaxseeds*	½
Hazelnuts*	8–12
Lentils	7
Macadamia*	2
Millet	5
Mung beans	8–12
Oats	6
Pecans*	6
Pine nuts*	2–4
Pistachios (shelled)*	2–4
Pumpkin seeds*	8
Sesame seeds*	8
Sunflower seeds*	8
Quinoa	4
Walnuts*	4
Wild rice	9

* After soaking, these foods usually need to be dried – see the instructions on the left.

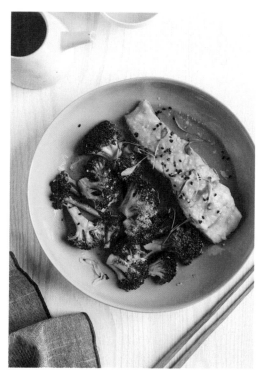

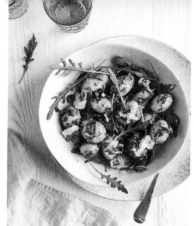

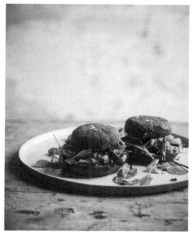

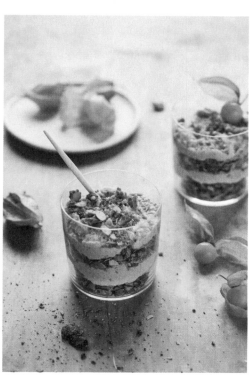

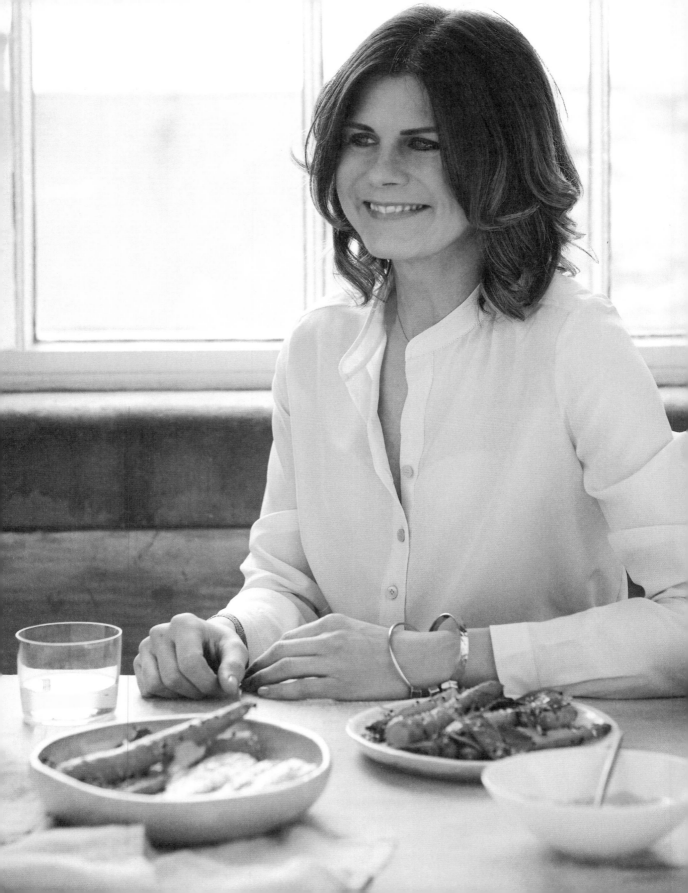

how to eat

EATING A MEAL may seem like a pretty average thing for most of us and we rarely think about what happens to the food after it leaves our fork. We take it for granted that our body will simply do what it needs to do to take care of that daily 'in and out' scenario. However, the process of digestion is far from average. In fact, it's pretty spectacular. Like a finely tuned orchestra, the gut plays a complex blend of roles: for example, activating hormones that manage our appetite and kick-start muscular movements; deploying substances such as enzymes to break down our food; and working diligently to absorb and assimilate nutrients that will be passed to other areas of the body. And let's not forget the trillions of microbes in the gut that get to work on the remnants, turning this veritable feast (well, to them at least) into essential anti-inflammatory substances and vitamins, among others. Suffice to say that what happens in the gut doesn't stay in the gut and the way our digestion functions has a much greater impact on our overall health than you might imagine.

a road map through digestion

In this chapter I will take you through all the twists and turns of our digestive system and explain how all these miraculous-sounding processes come together in perfect harmony. It's a fascinating process and should give you a newfound respect for your wondrous gut and its pivotal role in your health. Of course that respect should extend to the food on the plate in front of you, so at the end of the chapter you'll find some of my favourite recipes that support these processes and that will simultaneously have you heartily enjoying each and every bite. Buckle your seat belt and let's start our journey.

chew, chew, chew

Believe it or not, digestion starts in the mouth. We often forget this when we are furiously gobbling down food and barely chewing it, but this first step is critical. The act of mastication – the official term for chewing – activates saliva that, alongside other components, contains crucial digestive enzymes that help to break down our food. The combination of chewing and enzymes working on the food morsels breaks them down further so that digestion in the next part of the chain is easier. Breaking down food is a pretty demanding task for the body so taking the time and effort to chew enables enzymes to do their job properly, and allows the rest of the system to work much more efficiently.

If you have ever chewed a piece of bread thoroughly you will have noticed that it begins to taste very sweet. This is a result of the action of one of the main enzymes in saliva, salivary amylase, which has a pivotal role in breaking down carbohydrates into simple sugars. Some fat digestion also takes place in the mouth, via the enzyme lingual lipase, but this first part of the digestive process is mostly focused on dealing with the complex sugars and starches in carbohydrates. Depending on the type of carbohydrate, it may need to undergo a few rounds of 'dismantling', which is why proper mastication is so important.

Surprising as it may seem, you can alleviate some pretty unpleasant digestive symptoms simply by chewing properly. If large food particles move into the stomach and then enter the small intestine, this alone can result in bloating, cramping and gas, as a result of the resident bacteria getting to work on food that should have already been 'pre-prepared'.

When food is broken down adequately, it also makes it much easier for the body to absorb nutrients. This means it is not only what you eat that is important but *how* you eat. In fact, I would say it is better to eat a less nutritious meal and chew it properly than to scoff down a virtuous salad. If this isn't enough to encourage you to up the jaw action at meal times, spending longer over your meals also means you are likely to feel more satisfied because it allows time for the hormones that tell you 'enough is enough' to kick in. And that will make it less likely that you'll overeat or reach for that dessert.

eat well

Eating our food properly doesn't simply involve chewing and tasting it. To really connect with our food – and the process of digestion – we need to use all of our senses, which means fully immersing ourselves in the smell, texture and visual stimulation. And I don't mean from a tablet, computer or mobile screen! Our addiction to constant and multiple distractions has meant that meal times are often seen as an inconvenient necessity and are rushed through, when they should act as meaningful pockets of recovery in the day. Ubiquitous fast-food outlets and our high-speed lifestyles have led to us becoming a society of rapid eaters when really we need to backtrack a little and remind ourselves that meal times should be respected and enjoyed. Time spent over meals is still very much part of the culture in countries such as

tongue twister

Since digestion starts in the mouth and the tongue is an important part of that process, could it reveal more than you think about your digestive health? According to Traditional Chinese Medicine (TCM), the tongue can give clues to imbalances in the body. The theory is that the tongue acts as a mirror of the digestive system, reflecting such things as toxicity in the gut, malabsorption of nutrients or simply a weaker system overall. Modern medicine might not recognise the diagnostic usefulness of the tongue to the same extent but, nevertheless, a doctor will often look into the mouth for certain clues that may lead to further investigation. For example, a bright red tongue can be associated with B_{12} or iron deficiency.

So what does the perfect tongue look like? Think pink with a light white coating. According to TCM, a tongue colour that leans towards red or purple can indicate 'heat' in the body, possibly caused by hormonal changes, circulatory issues or inflammation. White, in contrast, is seen as a sign of deficiency, often of certain nutrients, particularly iron. A thick or very thin coating isn't ideal either as this can signal poor gut health. Yellow, grey or thick white are indicative of some kind of infection. And if the tongue is puffy with scalloped edges this can suggest nutrient deficiencies or poor detoxification.

Tongue scraping is considered an important part of oral hygiene in TCM. Advocates of this practice believe that daily tongue scraping gets rid of residual gunk and removes a lot of the bacteria hanging around in the mouth: there are 800 or so species in there, after all. The tongue should ideally be scraped every morning (copper or stainless steel tongue scrapers apparently give the best results). I've tried tongue scraping and found it left me with a much cleaner and fresher palate. Although there is no scientific backing for the practice, poor oral hygiene can be linked directly to other digestive issues, so perhaps adopting the morning mantra of 'wake and scrape' might not be such a bad idea.

Spain, Italy and France. Perhaps that's one of the reasons why the Mediterranean diet has such positive health correlations.

Here are a few simple steps you can take to drop the 'inhale and go' approach to eating and adopt better habits. Putting this into practice is one of the most fundamental things you can do for better gut health, and it will allow you to really appreciate the delicious recipes in this book. You will soon notice that eating intuitively makes such a positive difference.

- Respect your food. Eat it on a plate, with cutlery, sitting down (not standing by the fridge, your phone in one hand so that whatever you are eating is gone before you know it).

- Before you launch into your meal, pause and engage with what you are doing. Be present with the food that is in front of you. Too many of us mindlessly shovel it in while writing an email/sending a text/listening to a podcast … You get the picture.

- Take the time to really immerse *all* your senses in the food you are about to eat – the smell, the look and even the way it makes you feel.

- Taste your food. That means savouring the flavours and textures and noticing how they are released.

- Chew, chew, chew. Get those teeth and that jaw working. Aim for 30 chews per bite. You might find this tough to start with but practice makes perfect.

- Swallow and enjoy your food for a brief moment before taking your next bite.

- Stop eating when you are full, not when you have cleared all the food that's in front of you. Listen to your body.

the churner

When your food is ready to be swallowed, it is the job of a very clever organ called the oesophagus to send the chewed ball of food – the bolus – from the mouth to the stomach (or, as I like to think of it, the churner), where it meets a pool of gastric juices.

Unlike the mouth, which houses a huge diversity of bacteria, the stomach needs to sterilise a lot of potential pathogens to stop them moving further down your gut (think of it as the gatekeeper to the rest of the digestive system). It does this by releasing gastric juices – primarily hydrochloric acid – from parietal cells in the stomach. This creates a highly acidic environment with a very low pH. Think of battery acid and you get the picture.

The stomach needs to be highly acidic to stop disruptive microbes in their tracks and prevent them from migrating into areas lower down the gut, where they could create a whole host of nasty symptoms and potentially serious infections. Adequate levels of acidity in the stomach are also necessary to begin the process of digestion, especially of proteins, as this is where they are principally digested. Protein digestion is assisted by an enzyme called pepsin, which is secreted by cells in the stomach and starts to be activated upon mixing with the acidic gastric juices. The result of all this action is that proteins are broken down into smaller components, amino acids, that we can utilise for lots of vital processes around the body.

Unlike the mouth, the stomach needs to sterilise a lot of potential pathogens to stop them moving further down your gut (think of it as the gatekeeper to the rest of the digestive system).

Well that's how it *should* work. The problem is that in many cases the pH of the stomach is not acidic enough due to a deficiency in acid production. This can create just as much disruption to the gut as when acidity is too high – reflux and heartburn being the most common conditions at either end of the spectrum. Inadequate acid production can also lead to an overgrowth of bacteria in the small intestine, resulting in small intestinal bacterial overgrowth, or SIBO, which can then cause other gastrointestinal disorders. (We look at these issues in more detail in Chapter 3.)

Digestion in the stomach is further assisted by the contraction and relaxation of smooth muscles, guided by a number of hormones such as GIP (gastric inhibitory peptide), PYY and secretin, which work together to give a gradual and consistent movement. The resulting mush of what was the bolus now turns into chyme and is passed on, bit by bit, to the next part of the gut: the small intestine or, as I like to call it, the 'transporter'.

the transporter

This is where the process of digestion gets really serious. Having been chewed and churned thoroughly by the mouth and stomach, our 'morsel mush', now in the form of chyme, finds its way into the small intestine. This is where most digestive absorption takes place, and it is here that we assimilate the greatest amount of nutrients from our food. With its multi-folded surface, the small intestine does this with the help of tiny finger-like structures called intestinal villi. Each villi has multiple microvilli attached to it, and these project into the intestinal cavity. The microvilli are lined with cells that allow nutrients to be absorbed directly into the bloodstream, where they are transported to various parts of the body. The structure of the villi means that the surface area of the small intestine through which absorption can take place is vast, allowing a more efficient uptake of nutrients. Absorption in the small intestine is supported by a number of chemical substances, including digestive enzymes and bile acids, secreted by the pancreas, gall bladder and liver.

However, this entire absorption process relies upon the assistance of multitudes of microbes that reside in the small intestine. These microbes serve very important purposes. Firstly, they act like a checkpoint, managing and protecting the intestinal barrier to make sure that only substances that *should* be moving into the bloodstream get through. This is crucial for optimum uptake of nutrients and to avoid any potential inflammatory responses. In this protective function, these microorganisms also serve as the commanding force of the immune system. On top of all that, they support the muscular movement of the gut to ensure the chyme moves through the small intestine as smoothly and efficiently as possible (this is why chronic constipation can be indicative of a gut lacking in these helpful microorganisms).

Therefore, in a smoothly running digestive system, the small intestine should be the primary site of absorption – but things don't always stay on track. If there are imbalances, such as bacterial overgrowth or low reserves of digestive enzymes, they can compromise the ability of the small intestine to function optimally and, among other issues, affect the uptake of nutrients. (These are all crucial processes that we'll look at in more detail in later chapters.)

the transformers

By now I'm sure you're beginning to realise that absorption isn't just about what we eat but the many processes that are necessary in order to utilise the nutrients from our food. Certain substances manufactured by the body, such as the digestive enzymes mentioned above, are central to this, so let's look at where these guys come from.

To put it simply digestive enzymes work to break food down into smaller molecules so we can absorb them. They are found throughout the gut and in the form of amylase in the mouth and pepsin in the stomach. There are also enzymes embedded in the microvilli of the small intestine called 'brush border enzymes' that break down types of sugars and starches, including sucrose and lactase. And then you have the pancreas, which produces many more digestive enzymes found in pancreatic juice such as lipase for fat digestion and trypsin to support protein digestion. The pancreas is a highly skilled organ: it not only produces these enzymes but its juice also helps to reduce the high acidity of the chyme as it arrives in the small intestine. This is vital, as the small intestine prefers a more alkaline environment to do its work.

The pancreas is not alone in its crucially supportive role here; the liver and the gall bladder also have important parts to play in breaking down our food and absorbing nutrients. The actions of these three musketeers are in part managed and regulated by specific hormones, such as secretin and cholecystokinin (CCK). In addition to producing chemical substances such as digestive enzymes and acid-reducing sodium bicarbonate, the pancreas, liver and gall bladder all work to stimulate the secretion and release of bile.

Bile works almost like a detergent to break down fats which, in turn, allows for absorption of the fat-soluble vitamins from our food. Its other important function is to get rid of old red blood cells and excess cholesterol, which it dumps into the gut to be removed along with other 'waste' we don't need. The liver is the main organ in charge of the production of bile but it has a wingman in the form of the gall bladder, which helpfully stashes bile away for when these hormones kick in and tell it to release it into the gut. Low levels of bile can result in poor fat metabolism, indicated by light coloured stools. The causes of this can be structural, such as blocked bile ducts (which

requires medical intervention), or it could be that the flow of bile is simply on the sluggish side. Bitter foods such as artichoke have been shown to help stimulate the production of bile and some people swear by hot water with lemon juice first thing on waking. There's no research on this that I'm aware of, but getting into the habit of having water first thing is generally good for the gut, as it has thirsty work to do.

The role of the liver is paramount for digestion. As well as being key to the production of bile, it converts nutrients in our food into readily available materials and detoxifies harmful substances that we may have ingested. It stores glucose, the body's preferred energy source, as glycogen, so it is ready to be used when needed. It also has a 'bank' of vitamins and minerals that include vitamins A, D, E, K and B_{12}, as well as iron and copper minerals, so that the body has access to a constant supply. Moreover, the liver produces many of the chemical substances we need to function. And in any given second it is orchestrating hundreds of processes, including managing nutrients, toxins, enzymes, hormones, amino acids, drugs, energy production and metabolic compounds. You name it and the liver is working on it! It also has an incredible ability to regenerate and repair itself, which is reassuring, given all the responsibilities it has.

the terminator

Once the broken-down chyme leaves the small intestine it enters the large intestine, or colon, with very little 'food' left other than what cannot be absorbed. You could think of the large intestine as the waste disposal unit of the gut (I think of it as the terminator). It's certainly where we get rid of stuff that we don't need.

But amid this trash is treasure. While our body cannot break down food sources such as fibre, these leftovers provide a welcome meal for our microbes, so the colon is where bacteria really have a party.

In this part of the gut we can expect to find numbers of microorganisms into the trillions. This is their predominant turf and they are largely responsible for many of the digestive processes that happen in the colon. Eagerly awaiting fibrous food sources, these bacteria in turn feed cells in the colon with their waste products, having fully digested what they need. For example, short-chain fatty acids such as butyrate are essential energy givers for the cells in our colon and we depend largely on bacteria to make them. The colon is also where bacteria make many of the nutrients that are necessary for our bodies to function. We'll look at the roles these microorganisms play in more detail in the next chapter but suffice to say that without these multitudes of bacteria we would be in big trouble.

While the stomach and small intestine work intensively so that food passes through fairly quickly, in anything between six and eight hours for most people, the colon is slower because the bacteria need time to work on the undigested leftovers. That's why it's been suggested that having adequate breaks between our meals, essentially fasting periods, is probably a good idea to allow these microbes to get busy. Studies show that some methods of fasting are linked to an improvement in the balance of bacteria in the gut, and a number of other health markers (more on this in Chapter 10).

At this point in its journey our food has been subjected to chewing, churning, mixing, manufacturing and eventually to the final part of the journey, ready for its merry end in the toilet bowl. All being well, this should involve a daily visit, but don't panic if you are not that regular. It doesn't mean your body is more 'toxic', it may simply be that your bowel is a bit more relaxed when it comes to elimination. (We'll look at this topic in Chapter 3.)

the finale

So, having gone through all the nooks and crannies and a final bacterial swansong, our road trip of the mechanics of digestion is at an end. I'm sure that you now have much more respect for the multitude of processes that happen every time you dig into the plate of food in front of you. However, this chapter has simply set the scene, as there are many factors that influence how effectively we absorb our food and the way in which this magic happens. We'll look at these in the forthcoming chapters.

This chapter wouldn't be complete without a selection of tasty recipes containing some of the foods that can help the gut perform at its best. These are the ones that you should start to add to your diet more regularly, and I hope these recipes will inspire you to do that. Try my moreish Broccoli, Almond and Artichoke Dip (page 29) or my go-with-everything Watercress Pesto (page 28). Or, if you're looking for something sweet for breakfast that has bountiful digestive benefits, you'll love my Baklava Breakfast Parfait (page 27).

And of course, once you have made these delicious dishes, don't forget to savour and appreciate them wholeheartedly, taking time over your meal and chewing well. Your gut and the trillions of microbes that nourish and support you will certainly appreciate it.

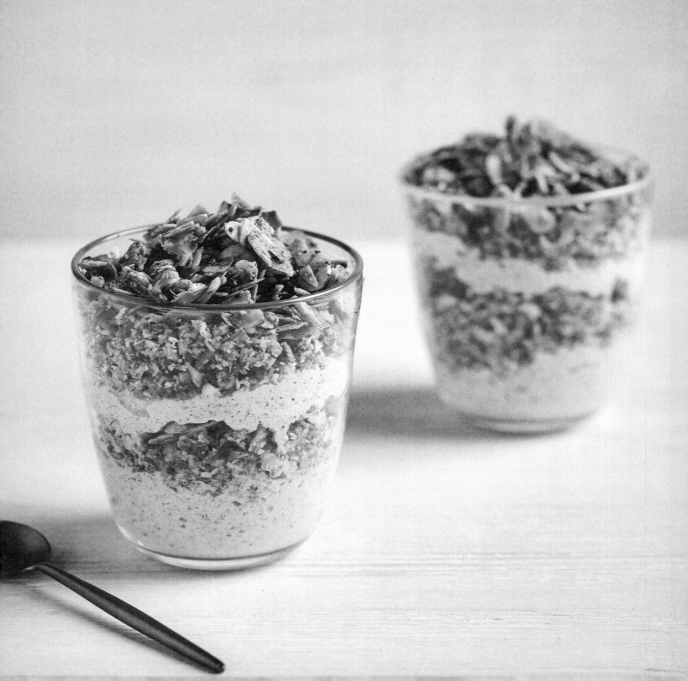

baklava breakfast parfait

I love baklava with a fresh mint tea, so I wanted to create the same flavours in this breakfast parfait. What's really great about this is that most of it is prepared in advance. You will need to 'activate' your pistachios and almonds by soaking them (see page 16) and this must be done at least 24 hours in advance, but you can make bigger batches and store them ready to use in other recipes or to eat as a snack. You can also prepare the 'phyllo' layer and the yogurt in advance. If these three elements are to hand then you only need to make the baklava filling in the morning and that takes all of about 10 minutes flat.

This moreish brekkie has gut friendly stamped all over it, right from the prebiotic pistachios through to the raw honey that help to feed and support our beneficial bacteria, along with myriad digestively soothing spices. Most importantly it's delicious and satiating and will see you through until lunchtime.

serves 2

'phyllo' layer
45g flaked almonds, toasted
20g coconut chips
1 tablespoon coconut oil, melted
½ teaspoon ground cardamom
½ teaspoon ground ginger
1 teaspoon ground cinnamon

baklava filling
20g ground flaxseed
1 tablespoon coconut flour
50g activated shelled pistachio nuts (page 16)
30g activated almonds (page 16)
1 teaspoon rose water
2 tablespoons raw honey
20g desiccated coconut
Pinch mineral-rich salt
Seeds from 1 vanilla pod

pistachio probiotic 'yogurt' (page 54)

First, make the phyllo layer. Preheat the oven to 150°C/ Gas 2. Line a baking tray with baking parchment. In a bowl, combine the flaked almonds and coconut chips with the coconut oil, cardamom, ginger and cinnamon. Place on the lined baking tray and bake for 15 minutes. Leave to cool for around 10 minutes. If making this in advance, transfer to a sealable jar or pot and store in the fridge.

To make the baklava filling, put the flaxseed, coconut flour, pistachios, almonds, rose water, honey, coconut, salt and vanilla into a food processor. Pulse briefly to break down into smaller sticky chunks.

To assemble, put 2 tablespoons of Pistachio Probiotic 'Yogurt' into two glass tumblers, then add 4 tablespoons of the baklava filling, then cover with a layer of the phyllo mix. Repeat to make another layer.

watercress pesto

This pesto is a firm fave of mine as it goes with everything! Spread on sourdough, mix through warm vegetables or serve as a side to some grilled organic grass-fed meat. It's also perfect in my Green Eggs and Ham recipe (page 132). Watercress is excellent for helping support natural detoxification and garlic could almost be considered a natural antibiotic. Also, like many bitter foods, watercress helps to stimulate gastric juices for better digestion. Soaking the nuts helps your body to absorb all their nutritional benefits (see page 16), and also improves the texture of the pesto.

makes 200ml (serves 4–5)

30g pine nuts, soaked for 2 hours
65g cashews, soaked for 2 hours
50ml extra virgin olive oil
1 garlic clove, peeled
Generous pinch mineral-rich salt
Generous squeeze fresh lemon juice
2 generous handfuls watercress (chuck in the stalks as well)

Drain the nuts and rinse thoroughly with filtered water. Put all of the ingredients into a food processor and blend until evenly mixed; this shouldn't be too smooth. Transfer to a sealable glass or ceramic container and place in the fridge. This will keep for up to 3 weeks.

tip

You can always sub in rocket for the watercress – it'll provide similar digestive benefits.

broccoli, almond and artichoke dip

Broccoli and artichoke are a fantastic pairing, taste and nutrition wise. In this partnership broccoli provides specific compounds that support natural detoxification, and artichokes, being bitter, can help stimulate bile for better digestion. The particular compounds in broccoli also assist our microbes in their metabolic activity as well as helping fight against pathogenic bacteria in the gut, keeping it a harmonious and happy environment. This dip is delicious on my Super Seed Bread (page 157) as a side to a soup, or with scrambled eggs in the morning. Buying artichokes precooked in a glass jar is ideal: you avoid the chemicals that can be present in some canned foods and it saves a lot of time too.

makes approx. 300g (4–5 servings)

1 medium head broccoli
1 garlic clove, peeled
120g cooked and drained artichoke hearts from a glass jar
½ teaspoon dried rosemary
4 tablespoons fresh lemon juice
½ teaspoon mild yellow mustard powder
50ml extra virgin olive oil
1 tablespoon almond nut butter
¼ teaspoon mineral-rich salt
Generous pinch black pepper

Preheat the oven to 200°C/Gas 6. Line a baking tray with baking parchment. Cut the broccoli into small florets and place on the lined tray, along with the garlic. Roast for 15 minutes.

Transfer the broccoli and garlic to a food processor and add all of the other ingredients. Process for a few minutes until you get a smoothish texture. Transfer to a sealable glass or ceramic container and place in the fridge. This will keep fresh for up to 3–4 days.

beetroot and goats' cheese stacks with hemp pesto and butterbean mash

Unpasteurised goats' cheese is packed with natural probiotics; it goes beautifully with the sweet taste of beetroot, which is an excellent source of fibre and antioxidants that support the beneficial bacteria in the gut. In a twist on classic pesto I've used hemp seeds instead of pine nuts. These creamy seeds have a perfect ratio of omega 3 to omega 6 essential fatty acids, which makes them a great plant-based natural anti-inflammatory. I use garlic and onion powder in my mash as they help to give a creamy texture, but feel free to use the fresh alternatives.

serves 2 (with extra pesto)

2 medium beetroots

50g unpasteurised soft goats' cheese, cut into thin slices

Extra virgin olive oil to drizzle

Herbs to garnish

hemp pesto

65g cashews, soaked for 2 hours

1 handful fresh basil leaves

25g shelled hemp seeds

50ml extra virgin olive oil

4 tablespoons apple cider vinegar

1 garlic clove, peeled and finely chopped

Pinch mineral-rich salt and black pepper

butterbean tarragon mash

150g cooked butterbeans (see tip)

¼ teaspoon garlic powder (or ¼ clove fresh garlic)

½ teaspoon onion powder (or 1 finely chopped spring onion)

4 tablespoons chopped fresh tarragon

1 tablespoon fresh lemon juice

2 tablespoons extra virgin olive oil

Pinch mineral-rich salt

Wash the beetroot and place in a steamer for 45 minutes to 1 hour or until cooked through. Remove from the heat, leave to cool slightly and then peel away the skin. Slice into 1cm slices (each beetroot should make approximately six slices) and put to one side.

While the beetroot is cooking, make the pesto and mash.

To make the hemp pesto, drain the soaked nuts and rinse with filtered water, then place all the ingredients in a food processor and pulse until blended but not too smooth. Put into a sealable glass or ceramic container. Rinse the processor.

To make the butterbean mash, place all the ingredients in the food processor and blend until you have a mash-like texture.

To assemble, start with a beetroot slice, add a thin slice of goats' cheese and a generous teaspoon of pesto; stack another beetroot slice on top and repeat the process, finishing with a slice of beetroot on top. There you have your stack. Repeat this same process to make more stacks. Serve a generous dollop of the butterbean mash alongside. Finish with a drizzle of olive oil over each stack and garnish with fresh herbs.

tip

To cook the amount for this recipe you will need 50g dried beans that have been soaked, drained and thoroughly rinsed. Put them in a saucepan with 250ml filtered water. Bring slowly up to the boil for 10 minutes, skim off the froth and then simmer gently for around 40 minutes.

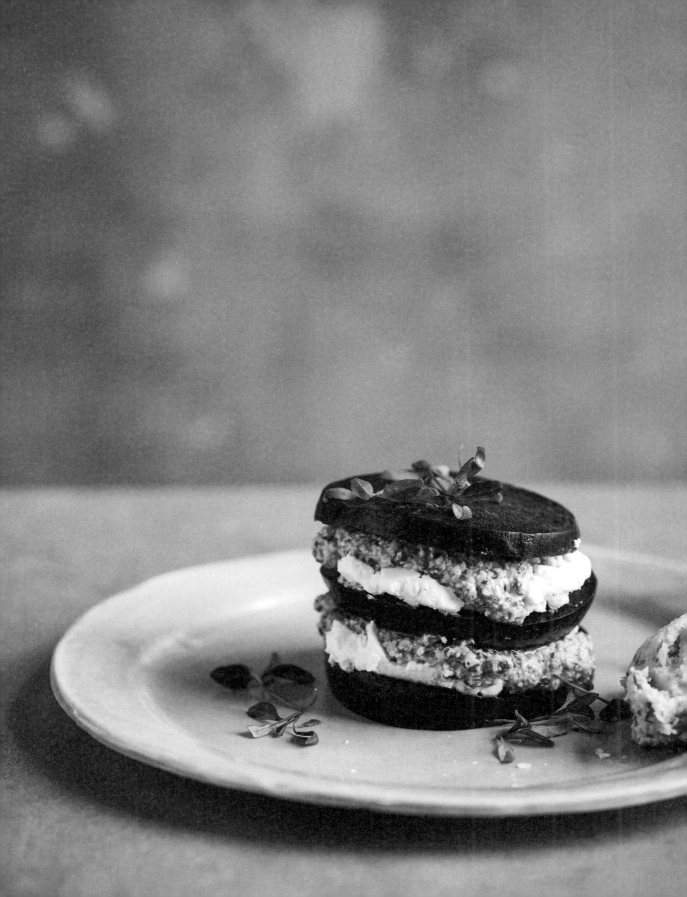

courgette, thyme and goats' cheese fritters

These are easy, quick and super satisfying. If you like, you can make up a double batch and take some to work with you the next day. My recipe uses coconut flour that not only gives a great taste but also supports those guts that are sensitive to gluten or other grains and is useful if you are doing an elimination diet. Feel free to experiment with other gluten-free flours such as buckwheat or quinoa. The unpasteurised goats' cheese adds a rich flavour and is generally more digestion friendly. These fritters are great with a green side salad and sweet potato wedges.

serves 2 (makes 6 fritters)

2 courgettes (approx. 300g), roughly chopped

1 organic free range egg, beaten

1 tablespoon apple cider vinegar

2 teaspoons chopped fresh thyme

1 teaspoon onion powder

¼ teaspoon garlic powder

50g ground almonds

20g coconut flour

30g unpasteurised soft goats' cheese

¼ teaspoon mineral-rich salt

Couple pinches black pepper

2 teaspoons organic unsalted butter or ghee

Extra virgin olive oil to drizzle

Put the courgettes in a food processor and pulse until broken down into small chunks. Transfer to a large bowl. Add the egg and all of the other ingredients, except the butter or ghee and olive oil. Mix thoroughly until you have a thick, dough-like consistency.

Take around 2 tablespoons of the mixture (about the size of a golf ball), roll into balls and then flatten to 2–3cm thick.

Heat a frying pan on a medium heat, add the butter or ghee and once melted add the fritters to the pan. You might need to cook them in two batches. Cook for 2–3 minutes on each side until they are golden brown and serve drizzled with a touch of olive oil.

trout, mint and pea rocket salad with almond tartare sauce

Trout can often be overlooked in favour of salmon but it ranks up there as one of the highest sources of healthy omega 3 essential fatty acids. When buying fish, always look for the blue MSC label, which means it comes from a sustainable source. For this salad I've added mint and peas to give it a fresh and vibrant hit. Mint is anecdotally a natural relaxant and is said to help digestion. I've also created a tartare sauce based on almond nut butter. I've used a white one for texture and colour, but you can use any type. Shop-bought sauces often contain hidden ingredients that are not always so kind to the gut.

serves 2

50g frozen garden peas

1 teaspoon organic unsalted butter or ghee

2 rainbow trout fillets, approx. 125g each

2 generous handfuls rocket

1 handful fresh mint, roughly chopped

1 tablespoon extra virgin olive oil

Generous squeeze fresh lemon juice

Pinch mineral-rich salt

tartare sauce

2 tablespoons white almond nut butter

2 tablespoons drained capers, finely chopped

3 tablespoons unpasteurised gherkins, finely chopped

3 tablespoons finely chopped fresh parsley

1 teaspoon onion powder

Generous squeeze fresh lemon juice

1 tablespoon extra virgin olive oil

Pinch mineral-rich salt

Pinch black pepper

Cook the peas by steaming or boiling for 5 minutes. Rinse through with cold water to stop the cooking process and place in a bowl to one side.

To make the tartare sauce, put all the ingredients in a bowl and stir to combine. Add filtered water to thin to a creamy consistency.

Heat the butter or ghee in a large frying pan on a medium heat. Add the trout fillets, skin side down, and cook for about 2–3 minutes, then turn and cook on the other side. Once cooked, remove from the pan and place on a chopping board or plate to cool.

Put the rocket, chopped mint and peas into a large bowl. Carefully flake the trout flesh (not the skin) into the salad, then add the olive oil, a squeeze of lemon juice and a pinch of salt and stir well to combine.

Divide between two plates and top with a tablespoon each of the tartare sauce.

miso cod with wasabi broccoli

Miso has been a traditional part of Japanese cuisine for over a thousand years; it is made from fermented soya beans. Like all fermented foods it is an excellent source of beneficial bacteria for the gut. The sweet white version is made with fermented rice as well as soya beans and works particularly well with white fish. Look for Atlantic cod with the MSC logo, which means it is sourced sustainably. Coconut aminos is an excellent alternative to soy sauce and is naturally sweet and gluten free, so it's an ideal replacement if you have an allergy to soya. If you want to make this a heartier meal, serve it with some soba (buckwheat) noodles.

serves 2

1 medium head broccoli

2 tablespoons unpasteurised sweet white miso paste

2 tablespoons sake

1 tablespoon coconut aminos

2 Atlantic cod fillets, approx. 150–200g each

1 tablespoon organic unsalted butter or ghee

1 garlic clove, peeled and cut into fine slices

¼ teaspoon wasabi powder

1 tablespoon sesame seeds

Preheat the oven to 180°C/Gas 4. Line a baking tray with baking parchment. Cut the broccoli into bite-size florets and place on the lined tray.

Mix the miso paste, sake and coconut aminos together in a small bowl. Place each cod fillet on a piece of baking parchment and spread the miso mixture evenly over the fish. Carefully wrap the paper around the fish to make a parcel and seal by folding over the ends so the miso mix doesn't run out the sides. Place the fish parcels on another baking tray and place both trays in the oven for 18 minutes.

Leave the cod to rest for a few minutes while you finish the broccoli.

In a shallow pan, heat the butter or ghee, add the garlic, broccoli and wasabi and stir-fry for 3 minutes.

Divide the broccoli between two plates and place the cod alongside. Garnish with the sesame seeds and pour over the juices from the cod parcels. Best enjoyed with chopsticks and a glass of sake on the side.

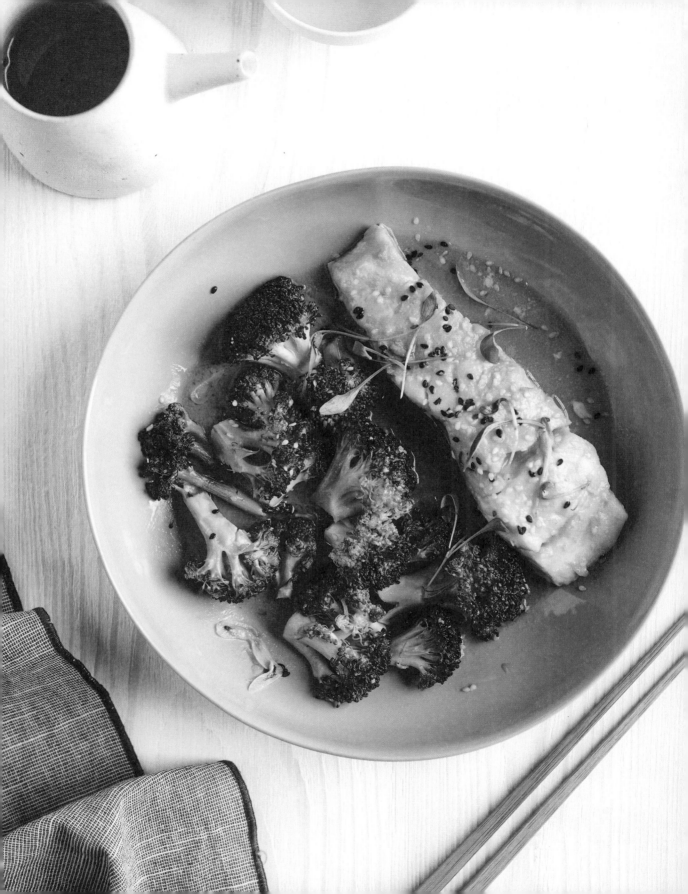

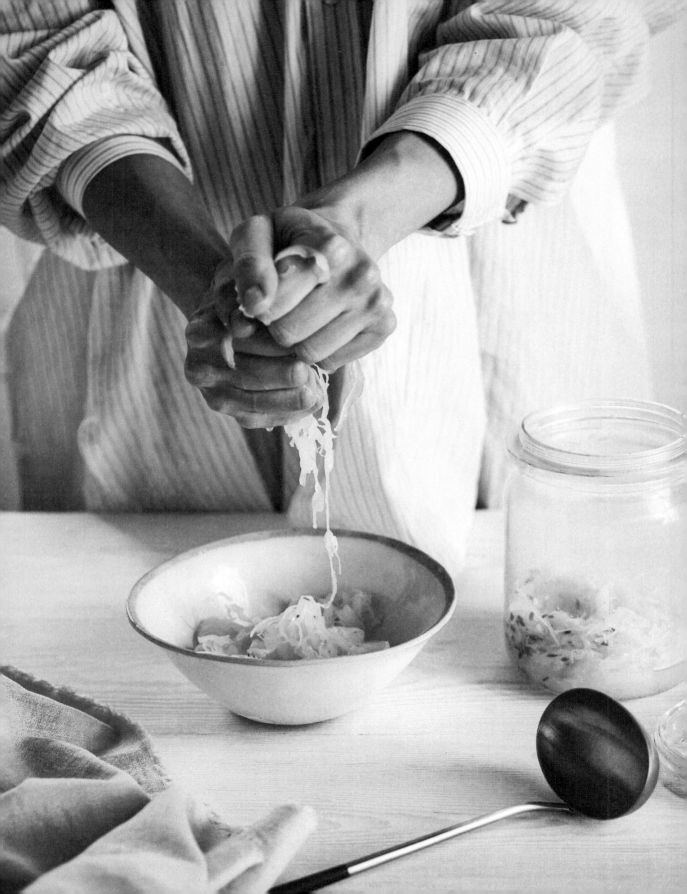

CHAPTER

2

the wonderful world of microbes

OK SO NOW we are going to get down and dirty. Yes I'm talking about the trillions of bacteria that reside in our gut. This chapter is all about delving a whole lot deeper into the gut and that starts and ends with the bacteria that reside there, collectively known as the 'microbiome'.

The very word 'bacteria' may have you swiftly reaching for the anti-bacterial spray to obliterate any and all of them. However, you will soon realise that not all these microorganisms are 'bad' and that in our current frenzy for all things anti-bacterial we are likely to be wiping out some that may be key players in our gut and our overall health. For sure, there are some bacteria that we could consider as generally having a positive effect on our gut and some that are

more negative, but to label them as 'good' or 'bad' is misleading, since nature is much more complicated than that. I prefer to describe them as disruptive and beneficial, as this recognises that both are on a continuum and it is only when the numbers of disruptive bacteria increase markedly that issues arise.

It is crucial to recognise when the balance in the microbiome has shifted in this way because it may potentially signal that your gut has become a stomping ground for more of these disruptive microorganisms to take precedence. Understanding how to address this is a critical part of getting your gut on the road to optimum health, so we'll look at how to do that in this chapter. We'll also examine the extent to which having a strong and robust gut depends on supporting our resident beneficial microbes, and the factors that can help your beneficial bacteria to thrive, as well as those that compromise their survival. This will enable you to cultivate and tend to your own inner ecosystem or, as I like to call it, your gut 'garden' and to follow my Weed, Seed and Feed programme at the end of the chapter.

Food really is the main 'fertiliser' for your gut microorganisms so I'll explain what is meant by probiotic and prebiotic foods and help you to introduce them into your everyday cooking repertoire with a collection of fun and delicious recipes, including my traditional family sauerkraut and an easy-peasy kefir. You'll also find some rather more unusual ones to tickle your palate, such as a mouthwatering Tempeh Reuben on Sourdough (page 61) and delectable Tiger Nut Macaroons (page 66). These are all foods that will not only have you licking your lips – your microbes are going to gobble them up with delight too. So without further ado, let's delve into the wonderful world of microorganisms.

the gut microbiome

We are more bacteria than we are human. That might sound like something out of a weird sci-fi movie, and it is certainly a strange concept to grasp, but, as I pointed out in the introduction, recent stats put the ratio of bacteria to human cells in the body at an average of around 1.5:1. Each and every one of us houses trillions of bacteria and for most of us up to 30–40 species. Between them they are thought to contribute a mind-blowing 8 million genes – a number that dwarfs our mere 22,000.

These incredible microorganisms are thought to have existed around 3.5 billion years ago but, surprisingly, the science on this stuff is fairly recent. It wasn't until the seventeenth century that we really started to understand more about bacteria and only in the twentieth century that probiotics were discovered. The more we uncover about how significantly these microorganisms influence overall health and wellbeing, the more we realise how much there is still to unravel. So far, scientists have merely scratched the surface when it comes to understanding this vast microbial kingdom.

from the beginning

Our intimate relationship with these microorganisms is a lifelong one that starts the moment we are born. Until we reach our birthday, the womb provides a sterile environment, but once we make our way into the world through a natural birthing process we are met with a host of microbes that give our gut the best possible start.

Babies who enter the world via a natural birth are inoculated with bacteria from their mothers' microbiome during labour. The bacteria from their mother's cervix and vagina begin to cultivate as soon as the baby leaves the birth canal, laying the foundations for their immune system. Many C-section babies, in contrast, don't receive their mother's resident 'population' and are likely to gain their first 'suitors' in the guise of microbes from the skin of the surgeon and nurses. As a result, such babies can have a less diverse microbiome, which may impact on how their immune system develops; for example, they may be at increased risk of atopic conditions such as asthma later in childhood.

These bacteria continue to flourish into early infancy through breast feeding, when babies gain further microbial diversity. Breast milk is therefore very important from a gut perspective. This is a crucial time in the shaping of the landscape of our gut and a lack of microbial diversity in these formative years can often be linked to gut-related health issues much later in life.

While how we were born and whether or not we were breast fed are important factors in shaping our microbiome, our intake of nutrient-dense foods during infancy is arguably the most important determinant of microbial diversity in the gut. And a diverse microbiome equals a strong and healthy gut. Exposure to as many different foods as possible during weaning is therefore ideal. By the time we reach the age of three to four our gut is said to have fully matured, so it is important to recognise how significant these early exposures are in establishing a healthy microbiome. We really do become what we eat.

but why are bacteria so important?

The role of bacteria in our health is one that is intrinsic and far reaching. Without them we would literally cease to exist. Having a healthy microbiome is essential for many reasons. Often we think of bacteria as being a bit alien to us, but they exist in every single cell of the body and make up between 1 and 3 kilograms of our entire weight. Some experts consider the microbiome an organ in its own right because of the many complex and crucial processes that gut bacteria perform. Certainly the constant communication and genetic 'chatter' of bacteria is felt throughout the body, from digestion through to hormones, neurotransmitters, detoxification, immunity and even weight management.

Let's look at the many positive roles of gut bacteria in more detail.

1. They're givers

Beneficial bacteria help produce and assist in the uptake of essential nutrients and other substances from the food we eat. While most nutrient absorption takes place in the small intestine, as I pointed out in the previous chapter, it is in the colon where bacteria really get to work. These bacteria use a surprising repertoire of enzymes to ferment and essentially 'eat' certain types of soluble dietary fibre that we cannot digest. This type of fibre – found in the cellular walls of some plants, fruits and seeds (for example, sweet potatoes, bananas, apples and flaxseed) – dissolves in water and, when fermented by the bacteria, creates a gel-like substance that helps support easier bowel movements. This process of transformative fermentation also provides us with small molecules that can be used by our cells for energy, and it is thought that between 10 and 15 per cent of our energy is obtained this way.

The most crucial element of this process is the production of short-chain fatty acids (SCFAs), the three main ones being butyrate, acetate and propionate. Short-chain fatty acids are the primary energy source for intestinal cells in the colon and have been shown to have many beneficial effects. For example, butyrate is the colon cells' main energy source and has shown promise in helping to manage various gastrointestinal diseases, including ulcerative colitis and Crohn's disease. Butyrate may also play a role in reducing inflammation, increasing the body's sensitivity to insulin (our blood sugar regulating hormone), and supporting immune responses. So the efficient production of short-chain fatty acids is critical not just for the gut but for overall health.

Bacteria do not simply break things down; they provide us with an abundance of nutrients, including the B vitamins biotin, thiamine, B_{12} and folic acid, as well as vitamin K. These nutrients are essential for processes such as producing energy, and for cardiovascular and bone health. Alongside this, they help with the absorption of minerals like calcium, magnesium and iron. And they can also synthesise certain essential amino acids (the building blocks of protein) so that, should reserves run low, we have a ready supply.

Recent research has also shown that gut bacteria can produce neurotransmitters such as serotonin, dopamine, acetylcholine and GABA (gamma-amino butyric acid), all of which affect our mood. In fact, they help to create an astounding 90–95 per cent of the body's total serotonin, which explains why there is often a strong correlation between digestive disorders such as IBS and depression. (You'll find more on the gut–brain connection in Chapter 5.)

2. Gut bacteria keep our immune army fit

Our microbiome has a vital role to play in providing the body with an internal army to fight off potential pathogens. Research has shown that without a plentiful microbiome, we would be much more susceptible to infections. The gut is where the external world comes into contact with our internal environment, mostly via the food and drink we consume, so our gut bacteria need to know how to react effectively and crowd out the microorganisms that may cause us harm. (It's a fascinating process, which we look at in Chapter 4.)

The gut is also a barrier that prevents toxins and other pathogens from finding their way into places that should be out of bounds, such as the bloodstream. Conversely, it allows through nutrients and other beneficial bacteria that have a role to play in keeping the system healthy and working efficiently.

3. They're liver supporters

The gut microbiome produces enzymes that are needed for the liver to transport certain substances out of the body. These enzymes help to break down compounds to be absorbed or excreted, including bile acids, cholesterol and hormones such as oestrogen. So you can start to see why having a gut microbiome that is working well can have a direct and positive influence on seemingly unconnected things, such as our cholesterol levels and hormonal balance.

4. Beneficial gut bugs help keep you trim

It is thought that imbalances in the gut microbiome can increase systemic inflammation in the body, which can contribute to weight gain. This has been linked to toxic substances, known as lipopolysaccharides (LPS), present in the cell wall of certain types of bacteria. It has been suggested that exposure to these LPSs triggers a heightened inflammatory state that seems to compromise metabolic processes and lead to weight gain. Furthermore, if our microbiome is compromised and we are not producing enough short-chain fatty acids (see point 1 above), this can also have a direct impact on our metabolism and appetite hormones, and hence our waistlines.

There is also research alluding to the role that gut bacteria play in appetite, and in the way we absorb and store calories as fat (covered in more detail in Chapter 9). Nevertheless, we know that bacteria in our gut like certain foods that help them to survive. This means that if they can find a way to influence what we eat, then they will stand a better chance of hanging out in the gut for the long term. It is therefore in their interest to send out cravings for these foods. This can often be the pattern in the case of chronic candidiasis (yeast overgrowth), where the urge to eat high-sugar foods can in some cases be insatiable. Now obviously this isn't good for the waistline, but at least you could partially blame your bacteria – and not your lack of willpower – for needing that large slice of cake! (If that sounds familiar then my Weed, Seed and Feed programme on page 46 can help you keep this kind of bacterial overgrowth in check and begin to quash those cravings once and for all.)

understanding the landscape of the gut

Now let's look at how we differentiate between generally beneficial bacteria and those that can create unpleasant symptoms. (If you'd like a brief overview on the composition of the gut microbiome, see the box below.)

what are gut microbes?

Microorganisms, or microbes, are microscopic organisms that cannot be seen with the naked eye. Those found in the gut come under the categories of bacteria, viruses, fungi, algae and protozoa. However, most microbes in the gut are from the bacteria kingdom, which is believed to feature anywhere up to 500 species (although we host closer to a modest 30–40). Within this gut bacteria kingdom there are thought to be four dominant 'phyla', or divisions – firmicutes, bacteroidetes, actinobacteria and proteobacteria, with the first two making up the larger proportion. The specific type and numbers of bacteria will be influenced by their microhabitat, which includes factors such as pH levels, exposure to nutrients and the body's secretions. The highest number of bacteria in the body reside in the gut, specifically the large intestine, or colon. Bacteria aside, the gut also houses other microbes such as fungi, including yeasts like candida, saccharomyces and Penicillium. Archaea is another type of microbial group in the gut and one that is important for the metabolic processes outlined earlier. It is these groups of microbes in the gut that are collectively known as the gut microbiome or microbiota.

Interestingly, recent research has shown that we have a genetic predisposition to one of three enterotypes (quite simply, a classification of gut microbiota): *bacteroides*, *prevotella* and *ruminoccucus*. It is thought that this is the reason why the uptake of nutrients can vary so much between individuals. For instance, those who have a *bacteroides* dominance tend to produce more vitamin C and B_2, whereas those leaning towards *prevotella* show increased amounts of B_1 and folic acid. This research is very much in its infancy but could potentially have compelling significance for how we support the gut on a case by case basis.

beneficial bacteria

These are sometimes referred to as 'probiotics' which essentially means pro-life. It is these beneficial microorganisms that enable most of the aforementioned processes to function at their best.

There are trillions of microorganisms in the gut, many of which have unique positive attributes, but for the purposes of simplifying this I'll focus on the two most widely researched families of beneficial bacteria – *Lactobacillus* and *Bifidobacterium*. Like other bacteria, within these categories is a vast number of species, sub-species and variant strains. The further down the intestine you go the more the numbers increase.

Lactobacillus should be most prevalent in the small intestine. They produce lactase and lactic acid, hence their name, which help to create an acidic environment in the gut. This environment crowds out alkaline-loving and potentially disruptive bacteria, as well as helping the body to absorb minerals such as calcium, copper, magnesium and iron. For example, *Lactobacillus acidophilus* (*L.acidophilus*), one of the most well-known *Lactobacillus* species, is a key player in maintaining the strength of the immune system and enabling proper nutrient absorption. Research has shown that *L.acidophilus* can also help relieve unpleasant digestive symptoms such as gas and bloating, and alleviate occasional diarrhoea.

The other family, *Bifidobacterium*, prefer to man the walls of the large intestine. Like *Lactobacillus*, they produce lactic acid which provides most of the energy for the cells that line and enhance the protective barrier of the gut. They are also largely responsible for the production of B vitamins and vitamin K. *Bifidobacterium bifidum*, for example, is one of the most dominant species in the large intestine. It supports the production of vitamins, helps beneficial bacteria to colonise the gut and inhibits the more harmful microorganisms.

As we age, overall levels of the *Bifidobacterium* family naturally decline so it is vital to feed them the nutrients that will help them thrive, such as soluble fibre and resistant starch, which we'll come on to shortly.

Another well-researched probiotic is a type of yeast called *Saccharomyces boulardii*, which has shown some promise with diarrhoea-predominant IBS and antibiotic-associated diarrhoea.

disruptive bacteria

Now let's look at the more 'unfriendly' microorganisms in the gut, which include pathogenic bacteria, certain types of fungi, such as *Candida albicans*, and parasites. These are the guys that can create havoc in the gut when they are left to proliferate and roam free. Think of it like a party: the odd uninvited guest isn't an issue but if too many party goers turn up it becomes more like a riot. The reality is that we will all 'flirt' with these types of bacteria at some time in our lives and it's important to note that you will never have a 100 per cent 'probiotic' gut. Aiming for an 85/15 split in favour of a healthy microbiome is a pretty good rule of thumb.

When the balance tips too far in favour of the more pathogenic bacteria, we start to see 'dysbiosis'. This means that the disruptive microbes outnumber and overwhelm the beneficial microorganisms and have a negative impact on the gut.

There are many reasons why dysbiosis can occur. Common factors include overuse of medication, particularly antibiotics; stress and the hormones produced during stress, which compromise the gut; a poor diet that includes a lot of processed foods, a low fibre intake, artificial sweeteners and high sugar consumption; slow gut motility; and, of course, direct exposure to specific pathogenic bacteria. However, there is rarely a single cause.

Symptoms of dysbiosis are not confined to the gut. Some pathogenic bacteria can adhere to the lining of the gut and from that vantage point secrete toxins that trigger a cascade of inflammatory responses that may be felt far from the gut itself. This kind of damage to the intestinal barrier does not simply cause inflammation, but also poor absorption and an over-sensitive immune system. This breakdown in the gut barrier has been referred to as intestinal permeability, or leaky gut, which we will focus on in Chapter 4.

If you suspect that all is not well with the bacteria in your gut, a functional stool test (see page 79) should reveal if there is an overgrowth of certain microbes in the gut. There are also some common signs and symptoms to look out for. These include (but are not exclusive to dysbiosis): erratic and urgent bowel movements, diarrhoea and/or constipation, sugar and carb cravings, recurrent yeast and urinary tract infections, skin conditions, poor sleep, IBS, bloating, undigested food in stools, indigestion, iron deficiency, hormone imbalances and fatigue.

feeding the beneficial bugs in our gut

Now that you understand the importance of maintaining the right balance of bacteria in the gut, let's look at how you can feed the beneficial bacteria the right types of gut friendly food so that they take precedence. Nourishing the beneficial bacteria with the correct sources of nutrients can alter the composition and diversity of the microbiota, allowing it to thrive and, in return, support and 'feed' us back tenfold. It's the perfect symbiotic relationship.

Taking in plenty of probiotic and prebiotic foods daily is an essential part of maintaining equilibrium in the gut. So what's the difference? Probiotic foods provide a direct source of beneficial microorganisms, whereas prebiotics feed bacteria so they are able to grow and thrive. Let's examine each in turn.

probiotic foods

Probiotic food sources include live, cultured yogurts, unpasteurised cheeses and fermented foods such unpasteurised kefir, kombucha, sauerkraut, miso and tempeh. The traditional methods used to preserve food, such as fermentation, will naturally produce high levels of *Lactobaccilli*, due to the lactic acid produced during this process, but they also provide other beneficial bacteria species. For example, half a cup of sauerkraut provides over a trillion probiotics, so including such probiotic foods daily in your routine is an essential part of keeping your 'ecosystem' nicely topped up. Plus they are super easy to make, as you'll realise when you start making your own kraut and kefir (see pages 58 and 153). You'll also see that in many of my recipes I add a touch of unpasteurised miso paste or cheese, which also provides a gentle boost of beneficial bacteria. Once you start eating these foods regularly they will simply become part of your routine.

It is then vital to support your resident beneficial microorganisms with their favourite food sources, so they can repopulate and ensure that the balance continues to swing in a favourable direction. This is where prebiotics come in.

prebiotic foods

Prebiotic foods contain a type of non-digestible fibre found in the cell walls of plants in the form of carbohydrates such as polysaccharides, oligosaccharides and resistant starches. Since the body is not able to digest these fibres they find their way intact to the large intestine, where the microbiota gobble them up for us. Essentially these foods provide nutrient fuel for the beneficial bacteria and work with them to retain balance and diversity in the gut. It's a happy and harmonious relationship.

Prebiotic foods include onions (raw or cooked), raw garlic, leeks, raw chicory root, raw asparagus, Jerusalem artichokes and unripe bananas. Some of these foods can be tricky to incorporate into your diet but it can be done. For example, try adding garlic at the end of cooking rather than at the start and using it raw in dips and spreads – something like my Watercress Pesto (page 28) works well. Thinly sliced raw asparagus and Jerusalem artichoke are delicious in salads. And ground chicory root is an excellent coffee replacement, so not only can you reduce caffeine consumption (if you drink a bit too much) but it gives a nice boost to the gut.

Bacteria particularly love resistant starch (RS). Like soluble and insoluble fibre, resistant starch moves through the digestive system largely untouched before it is fermented in the large intestine (hence 'resistant' starch). Intestinal bacteria ferment the resistant starch to produce short-chain fatty acids, such as butyrate, as mentioned earlier, and which we know to be intrinsic to a healthy gut. Butyrate production, in particular, is positively influenced by resistant starch and it has been shown that regularly ingesting this type of prebiotic has beneficial effects on the colon and can improve certain gastrointestinal conditions.

Resistant starch is found in foods such as cooked and cooled legumes and pulses, cooked and cooled white potatoes, sourdough, uncooked oats and unripe bananas. Potato salads (see my Punchy Potato Salad on page 62) and cold lentils stirred through salads are simple and easy ways to boost your levels of this beneficial prebiotic. One thing to note: go easy with prebiotic foods at first, particularly if you are someone who has a penchant for white refined foods, as there will be a sudden feeding frenzy among the bacteria and the resulting bottom burps won't be pleasant. Start slowly and gradually increase your intake.

anti-microbial foods

As well as including both probiotic and prebiotic foods in your diet, including plenty of natural anti-microbial foods can further help to retain equilibrium in the gut. These foods can help control the overgrowth of more pathogenic organisms and, in doing so, boost beneficial bacteria. Coconut oil is one such food. It has been shown to have anti-bacterial, anti-fungal and anti-parasitic properties and can easily be added to a smoothie, porridge or a stir-fry. Likewise garlic, ideally in its raw state, provides similar anti-microbial benefits. Fresh herbs such as oregano, thyme and rosemary can also help to support the microbiome (also see box page 47), and spices such as chilli, turmeric and cumin contain natural chemical 'defence' compounds. You will find many of these ingredients used liberally in my recipes.

to supplement or not to supplement?

There are many different probiotic supplements on the market but it is important to remember that our ancestors got their daily dose from cultured and fermented foods. Traditionally that was how we maintained a healthy gut, so ideally you should be doing this too, rather than relying solely on supplements. That said, probiotic supplements can help to support the health of our gut and inner ecosystem. But with so many options on the shelves, you need to know how to be discerning.

Many of the probiotic formulas on the market are at best less effective or at worst devoid of any benefits at all due to the formulation. This is because a lot of the commercially available probiotics are produced from milk in an aerobic environment (note: most of our bacteria is anaerobic). In addition, many of the strains included can be destroyed by stomach acid or bile salts before they reach the areas of the gut they are supposed to target, and, if they do get through, they fail to have real 'sticking' power so are just as quickly eliminated.

So, how do you choose the right supplement?

- Do your research. Any decent probiotic manufacturer should have some clinical research to support their products, so always check their credentials.

- Look for a diverse formula that contains multiple strains but don't be too focused on getting the widest number of strains. Quality over quantity is the rule of thumb.

- Look for the strains that survive the acidity of the stomach, adhere well to the gut wall and repopulate well once they arrive there. Current research highlights some of these, including species such as *bacillus subtilis*, *L.rhamnosus*, *L.Planatarum*, *B lactis* and *saccharomyces boulardii*.

- Look for a decent amount of probiotics in the formula. This is referred to in terms of CFUs (colony-forming units). Somewhere around the 10 billion mark is a good starting point but again don't fixate on the number, it really comes down to the quality and survivability of the probiotics you are taking.

- Don't assume that the ones that require refrigeration are always the best. Production techniques are developing rapidly in this area so it is not a hard and fast rule that you need to take these types of probiotics (although sometimes they are the most appropriate and effective).

- Target your probiotic for your specific needs. This is always going to be a more intelligent approach to supporting any kind of imbalance so it's worth doing a bit of research to get this right. As more and more research unfolds in this area, it is also possible to be prescriptive with your probiotic. For example *L.Planatarum* 299V has been show to affect iron absorption whereas *L. rhamnosus* GR-1 has been linked to improved vaginal health.

Eating probiotic and prebiotic foods will provide and nourish beneficial bacteria and this is where you need to start. It's not about 'jacking up' with tons of supplements. Commonly they can provide additional support in cases of dysbiosis or a compromised digestive system and to give your microbiome a well-deserved boost during the Weed, Seed and Feed programme.

Hopefully you now understand why it's so important to nourish your microbes. I've given you a lot of information to take in but gradually incorporating some of these simple daily habits can make a big difference. Kicking off your day with my Lip-Smacking Lucuma Smoothie Bowl (page 55) or Pistachio Probiotic 'Yogurt' (page 54) can get your beneficial guys off to a flying start. And even just a simple side of sauerkraut with poached eggs on sourdough at brunch is another way to give them a welcome boost. We all need to love and care for our beneficial bugs and that starts with the foods on the plate in front of you and some gentle tending to your own gut 'garden' from time to time. That's what my Weed, Seed and Feed programme is all about.

On page 258 you'll find a one-week menu planner to give you an idea of how to mix and match recipes while following the programme.

weed, seed and feed – your 30-day programme

Creating and maintaining a healthy gut and a flourishing microbiome starts with supporting your own 'ecosystem'. My Weed, Seed and Feed programme is the culmination of everything I've outlined in this chapter, and is designed to start you on a journey to rebalancing and healing your gut. It won't solve serious gut problems but if you are looking for a way to address some longstanding gut symptoms, it can be a great place to begin. Equally, those of you with no apparent tummy troubles can reap the benefits from giving your gut a bit of love and attention.

This isn't a detox or a diet. Instead think of it as kick-starting a lifelong approach to consistent good gut health. You'll find guidance on how to use elements of the programme at the end of the 30 days on page 53. I have also included a handy shopping guide on page 261 that you can refer to if there are any ingredients that you are unfamiliar with in the 'in' list (page 49) or the recipes.

The analogy of a garden really epitomises our gut on many levels. Think of the more disruptive bacteria discussed earlier as the weeds, the terrain of the gut as the soil, gut-supportive nutrients as the fertiliser and probiotic microorganisms as the seeds. Just as you wouldn't plant seeds in your garden without weeding and prepping the soil, you have to think about preparing the gut in the same way. You can't expect beneficial bacteria to thrive if they are overwhelmed by weeds. Following my three-step plan for 30 days can help give your gut the care and attention it needs in order to be vibrant and blooming.

weed

Weeding out disruptive bacteria and foods that may be causing warfare in your gut is the first step and should be followed throughout the 30 days. That means removing some of the possible dietary triggers that may be contributing to chronic inflammation, including refined sugars, commercial cow dairy products, soya and gluten. This is not to say all of these foods are 'bad' but if your gut is irritated, they can perpetuate the cycle of inflammation. This section of the programme is about stopping that cycle. Think of it as pressing a 'reset' button for your gut by removing certain foods from your diet.

the 'out' list...

The following foods should be removed from your diet during the programme.

commercial cow dairy

- **Avoid** all types of commercial cow milk, cream, cheese and yogurts. Lactose sensitivity can promote inflammatory responses but more often it's the processing that most of commercial dairy undergoes that can create digestive issues in some people (this is covered in Chapter 6). Note that unsalted organic or cultured butter and ghee contain very little to no lactose and some great saturated fats, so enjoy these in moderation.

- **Alternatives** Include small amounts of unpasteurised goat or sheep cheese or full fat organic sheep or goat yogurt, as these tend to be better tolerated and contain natural beneficial bacteria. Coconut yogurt can also work well and is completely dairy free. Nut-based unsweetened milks, such as almond, hazelnut, Brazil or cashew, can also be great

anti-microbial herbs

You may want to consider adding in a broad-spectrum concentrated anti-microbial herb, such as oregano oil, for the first 14 days of the programme. It can help with dysbiosis, but take it in small doses – it's potent stuff! (And make sure you get it from a reputable source and that it is pure, organic and wild.) Ideally, you would work with a practitioner who can run functional testing, such as a stool analysis, as this will give a more comprehensive overview of the microbiome and enable these to be addressed more specifically. However, as a general pathogenic 'hit man', oregano oil has shown some benefits. Anti-microbial herbs, when taken in a potent form such as oregano oil, will generally have a stronger effect on the overgrowth of bacteria than their food counterparts but, unlike the food, they should not be used on an on-going basis. In a short programme such as Weed, Seed and Feed, they can give an extra boost to the gut. See my resources section for more information on recommended stockists. Avoid oregano oil if you think you have any contraindications.

replacements for dairy (you'll find recipes for these on pages 150–151). Coconut milk is delicious if you need a denser, creamier taste or texture (it's also delicious in coffee). Kefir can be a great addition to your diet but go for homemade with organic full fat unhomogenised milk. Start culturing your own with the recipe on page 153.

grains

- **Avoid** foods that contain wheat, rye, bran, flour, bulgur and barley, which means most breads, bagels, crispbreads, cereals, pasta and crackers. Wheat and gluten sensitivity in particular can be problematic for a compromised gut, often because of the way the grain has been processed and/or prepared (we look at this in more detail in Chapter 6).

- **Alternatives** Use small amounts (a maximum of two to three servings per week) of gluten-free grains such as quinoa, buckwheat, gluten-free oats and amaranth. The important point is to *rotate* these grains and eat them in their most natural state, rather than buying processed, 'free-from' gluten substitutes. Ensure you properly prepare these grains by soaking or sprouting them so that they are more gut friendly (see page 16). Even with these gluten-free grains, try to stick to those two to three servings so you can minimise irritants to the gut. Swap regular flours for coconut, tiger nut, chestnut and ground almonds. Alternatively, make grain-free breads such as my Super Seed Bread (page 157), Broccoli and Walnut Bread (page 226) or Matcha Banana Bread (page 128). Cauliflower rice, which features in a few recipes, is also a great grain replacement. (Sourdough bread can be added in after the 30-day weeding phase, as the fermentation process it undergoes means the gluten is largely pre-digested and it's bursting full of natural probiotics, but during this period it should also be avoided.)

refined sugar

- **Avoid** sweets, cakes, cookies, ice cream, sugary cereals and granolas and fizzy drinks.

- **Alternatives** Avoid excessive amounts of the 'healthy' syrups such as agave, maple and brown rice. Instead, opt for small amounts of local raw honey (1 teaspoon per day). Make sure it is raw, though, as the refined stuff is really just sugar. Sugar in *any* form in excessive amounts can disrupt the microbiome. Have a look at some of my sweet fix options such as the Tiger Nut Macaroons (page 66) or my sugar free ice creams (yes, you read that right) on pages 183–186.

white refined carbs

- **Avoid** white bread, crisps, sugary cereals, pastries and chips. This 'beige buffet' has the same effect as sugar.

trans fats

- **Avoid** ready meals, ready-made sauces and condiments, low-fat foods, biscuits, margarine, fried fast food, takeaways and pizzas. If you can get it on speed dial then it should not be on the menu. These fats are a grenade for the gut and can create more systemic inflammation in the body. (See page 169 for details on why they are so harmful.)

alcohol

- **Avoid** all alcohol – it's only for 30 days! Once you've finished the programme it's fine, in fact healthy, to have the odd glass of good quality wine (see page 173), but when dealing with an inflamed gut, drinking alcohol is like putting fuel on the fire.

- **Alternatives** Try putting some mineral water flavoured with fresh lemon or mint into a wine glass and sipping from that. Sometimes it is the motion of lifting the glass that psychologically helps kick in those feelings of relaxation and reward. Find non-food related rewards that give you that high – taking a relaxing bath or listening to soothing music for example.

too much raw food

- **Avoid** eating too much raw food. It is energy dense but you need a pretty robust gut to break it down, so too much can be hard work when your gut is already struggling. Try to lightly steam your veggies as opposed to eating lots of them raw. However, it is important to include some raw food earlier in the day (when your digestion is more robust), such as a small side salad at lunch or some rocket with eggs in the morning.

junk soya

- **Avoid** soya milks, desserts, yogurts and meat substitutes – unless you make them yourself – as a lot of these products include added sugars and ingredients that can also create digestive symptoms.

- **Alternatives** Non-GMO tempeh and unpasteurised pure miso paste are the exceptions here as they are fermented from their original form. Non-GMO, plain organic tofu in small amounts is also fine – I have highlighted a couple of brands in the shopping list for you. Use tamari or coconut aminos as a replacement for soy sauce.

excess fruit

- **Avoid** eating too much fruit. Stick to one serving per day, such as an apple or pear, a small banana or a cup of berries. When we stop eating refined sugar, there's a tendency to overdo it with fruit. It's a healthier form of sugar than the white stuff but too much fruit still equates to too much sugar, natural or otherwise.

excess caffeine

- **Avoid** caffeine for a while if you are particularly sensitive to it and/or have high levels of stress. Otherwise, one cup of fresh coffee or caffeinated tea in the morning after eating is usually OK for most people.

- **Alternatives** Try using ground chicory for a similar flavour and a prebiotic boost. Organic, loose-leaf green tea is excellent and also supports natural detoxification processes.

chemical additives

- **Avoid** the artificial sweeteners, preservatives and emulsifiers that you generally find in processed food. If you can't pronounce the ingredient or don't recognise it as a genuine food source don't eat it.

the 'in' list...

Here's what you should be eating in abundance throughout the 30 days.

veggies

Go for as much variety as possible. Think diversity rather than focusing on the amount (although five to ten servings would be ideal). Eating lots of different coloured veg – the 'rainbow' as it is often called – provides a wider range of nutrients and supports the growth of multiple beneficial bacteria. In particular include the orange ones, such as carrot, butternut squash and sweet potato, as they are rich in beta-carotene (a type of vitamin A), which is crucial for the health of the gut. Always try to pair these with some kind of healthy oil to absorb this fat-soluble vitamin. Dark leafy greens are also excellent for their beta-carotene content and are brimming with B vitamins that will keep your energy levels buoyant. Cruciferous veggies such as broccoli, cauliflower and cabbage are also an excellent support for natural detoxification processes. Chucking veggies into a smoothie, making dips and soups are all easy ways to up your quota. Point to note: during this programme white potatoes should be eaten fully cooled after cooking, when the starch in them behaves very differently (so don't have them hot during this time).

omega 3 oils

Wild oily fish, organic grass-fed, free range or pasture-raised meat and poultry – and, for plant-based options, linseed/flaxseed and chia – all provide omega 3 oils (essential fatty acids that help to support anti-inflammatory processes). Typically we don't take in enough of these. Sardines are brilliant flaked through salads or paired with some sweet potato wedges and my Chipotle Red Pepper Dip (page 178). Or try my Wild Salmon with Roasted Carrots, Leaves and Miso Kefir Dressing (page 231).

healthy fats

Coconut oil, organic butter or ghee, avocado and coconut milk are all gut-supportive (you can read more about some of these in Chapters 8 and 9). Use cold pressed oils, such as extra virgin olive oil, for drizzling over food *after* you have cooked it, as most of them don't perform well at high temperatures and can have a negative health impact when exposed

to heat. Try to aim for a tablespoon of coconut oil every day, added to smoothies, pancakes or porridge for example, as it inhibits the growth of pathogens and yeasts.

raw apple cider vinegar

Anecdotally cider vinegar has been linked to supporting the balance of bacteria in the gut. Plus it's a good alternative to vinegars that contain sugar, as it's naturally sweet. Add to dressings for salads and veggies or just take a neat shot before your meals with a dash of filtered water if you're brave enough.

certified organic and spray free

Try to include as much certified organic and spray-free food as you can. Top of the list and non-negotiable should be your meat, poultry and eggs (which should also be free range and grass fed). Certain veggies and fruits tend to have higher pesticides than others so do a bit of research using resources such as PAN UK or EWG (see page 270) and then try to buy the worst offenders organically. Going to farmers' markets and speaking directly to the producers is a great idea and most will be transparent about the sprays that they use.

chewing!

As we saw in Chapter 1, if you are not chewing your food properly you are asking your gut to work that much harder further down the line, which can in itself create dysbiosis and affect absorption. There is little point putting in all these nutritious foods if you're not giving yourself the best possible chance of reaping the benefits.

fasting

Giving your gut adequate time to rest is a crucial part of nourishing it. That means leaving at least 4-5 hours between each meal. If you have eaten enough protein and healthy fat at each meal you shouldn't feel the need to snack in between. Moreover, time-restricted eating, which means leaving 12 hours from when you finish your evening meal to having breakfast, should be the aim during this programme and I would suggest retaining this pattern for the long haul. This is beneficial not only for your gut but also for your metabolism. The aim is to keep your meal times between a 12-hour window, so if you eat breakfast at 8am then aim to have finished your supper by 8pm.

seed

After 14 days of 'weeding' your gut should be a more welcoming home and the perfect environment for beneficial bacteria to thrive. At this point we can begin to 'seed' the gut with probiotics from natural sources and a good supplement. This will start to cultivate and support the growth of beneficial bacteria.

During this phase, include the following foods in your diet.

fermented foods

This includes unpasteurised (or raw) sauerkraut, kimchi and pure miso paste; also tempeh that is GMO free and unpasteurised kefir or unpasteurised goat and sheep cheese. These all provide trillions of natural probiotics. Go slowly if you are new to these foods but do try to incorporate at least one on a daily basis. My recipe for Sauerkraut (page 58) is a brilliant and tasty probiotic side dish for *any* meal, or make the Kefir on page 153, which you can include as part of your morning ritual.

probiotic supplement

A good probiotic supplement can help to bolster those beneficial microorganism numbers. Check out my shopping guide (see page 266) for recommendations but do your own research, too.

digestive enzymes

Many people have low levels of the digestive enzymes I discussed in Chapter 1. These are crucial for breaking down your food and low levels can also contribute to symptoms such as bloating, gas, IBS, constipation and diarrhoea. Partially digested food can also create inflammation in the gut, so taking enzymes as a supplement just before a meal may help to reduce this, and I would advise doing so throughout the 30 days to give your gut an extra boost. See page 266 for my recommendation. For natural digestive-enzyme-rich food sources that you should also include (even if you are taking a supplement) try fermented vegetables and raw honey (best eaten with other foods to aid digestion). In contrast, papaya, which also contains enzymes that assist with breaking down protein in particular, is better eaten 15–20 minutes before a meal. Try it as a nice warm up to your breakfast in the morning or add it to a small salad just before lunch.

vitamin d

It is also a good idea to check your vitamin D levels as this is a vital nutrient for the intestinal barrier. If you need to supplement then you can add this too (see page 266).

feed

While you are seeding the gut with probiotics it's also important to feed beneficial bacteria the right nutrients so they can continue to flourish. Some foods should be included regularly in the diet so you can continue to maintain homeostasis in the gut. This should be followed alongside the seeding phase and these foods should be included in your diet as much as possible beyond the programme itself.

prebiotics

Add prebiotic foods such as onions, raw garlic, leeks, Jerusalem artichokes and ground chicory, as well as resistant starch foods like cooked and cooled potatoes, unripe bananas and uncooked gluten-free rolled oats (ideally soaked). A simple breakfast of soaked oats blended with an unripe banana puree can give you an easy morning prebiotic boost or try my Lip-Smacking Lucuma Smoothie Bowl (page 55).

chicken soup for the soul (and the gut!)

I'm specifically referring to organic bone broth here, which contains amino acids such as l-glutamine, proline and glycine and is a direct source of collagen that can help to support the strength of the intestinal barrier. Aim for 250–500ml per day. Whether it's chicken, beef, pork, lamb or fish versions, they all contain the amino acids and nutrients to support the intestinal barrier. Bone broth is pretty easy to make yourself (see my recipe on page 57) but you can also buy it from a reputable source (see page 261). Add as a hearty base to soups, stews, sauces or warm it and drink on its own. If you are vegan or vegetarian, a broth rich in seaweeds such as wakame, plus green leafy veggies and pure miso paste can support collagen production and with a side of sauerkraut provide a hit of glutamine, one of the amino acids most closely linked to good gut health.

an apple a day

Lightly stewed apples provide a readily available source of fibre in the form of pectin, which helps to feed microbes in the gut and encourages the production of short-chain fatty acids such as butyrate, mentioned earlier. See page 111 for a delicious recipe with a honey kefir cream. Try to have one organic apple per day prepared this way.

don't forget your mind

A stressed mind leads to a stressed gut so feed your body with restorative activities. Creating day-to-day pockets of recovery in whichever way works best for you is super important; it could be making that regular yoga class a 'not to be missed' appointment or scheduling in breathing or meditation. The easiest and probably the most critical one is having meals in an environment conducive to 'rest and digest' without distraction – to better absorb the delicious and nutritious food that you will be eating and to allow the natural healing processes of the body to take full effect. It's also important to switch off blue light devices such as laptops, tablets and smartphones at least an hour before going to bed. This helps to support your circadian rhythms so you sleep better and it allows the body's overnight repair mechanism to kick in.

after 30 days

Having followed the programme for 30 days you should start to feel positive shifts in your gut. *But*, and this is a big but, everyone is different. Some people start to notice differences almost immediately and with others it takes a bit longer. It really depends on how much tending is needed for your own 'garden'. Regardless of this, the seed and feed recommendations are not something to abruptly drop after you finish the programme; far from it. Adopting a daily habit of eating fermented, probiotic and prebiotic foods is essential for ongoing optimum gut health.

You can start to reintroduce some of the foods in the 'Weed' section *slowly* once you have completed the 30 days, with the exception of the refined sugars, processed foods and trans fats, as these in excess are never going to be good for you or your gut. Just be mindful of the type of food you are eating and note where you might have reactions to certain foods that simply don't agree with you. It's not so much that you should never eat cow-dairy again but just be more discerning – go organic, unpasturised and unhomogenised where you can, and don't overdo it. Many of these 'trigger' foods are simply eaten in too great a quantity, too often. And, frankly, by the end of the 30 days you may not even crave some of the high sugar or junk foods that you once enjoyed. By supporting the gut you can also shift your taste buds.

The other great thing about this programme is that you can repeat it a couple of times per year to give your gut that extra boost when you need it. What's more, because this doesn't require any extreme measures, excessive supplementation or being overly restrictive, it is easy to follow, includes delicious foods and is suitable for pretty much everyone.

By practising your own personal 'horticulture' you'll realise the potential of your gut to blossom and you'll soon find that having healthier and happier digestion really is achievable … and enjoyable!

Note: *If for whatever reason you still feel that things haven't improved then seek the help of a nutritional therapist who can delve a bit deeper and tailor a programme to your needs. And if you think you may have any contra-indications, always check with your GP before starting any nutrition programme.*

pistachio probiotic 'yogurt'

This is pure heaven on a spoon. It reminds me a bit of the pistachio ice cream you can get at a traditional Italian gelateria but with a hint of sourness. And the best bit is it's great for the gut too. Soaking nuts allows the gut to better absorb the nutrients (see page 16). Adding kefir gives it that distinct yogurt taste due to the natural fermentation process, which also means it packs in tons of beneficial bacteria. I would advise that you use a powerful blender to get the smoothest consistency. This recipe goes beautifully with the Baklava Breakfast Parfait on page 27.

makes about 300g (one small pot)

100g shelled pistachio nuts, soaked for 2 hours

125g cashews, soaked for 2 hours

200ml dairy or coconut kefir (page 153)

Pinch mineral-rich salt

Seeds from 1 vanilla pod

Drain the nuts and rinse thoroughly with filtered water. Place in a high-speed blender with the kefir, salt and vanilla, then blend on the highest setting until smooth.

Pour into a glass or ceramic container and allow to cool. Cover with an airtight lid and store in the fridge. It will keep well for up to 3–4 days.

lip-smacking lucuma smoothie bowl

This breakfast bowl tastes just like caramel and it's a sweet treat for your gut microbes too. The caramel flavour comes from lucuma powder – the dried flesh of a fruit native to the Andes, which acts as a natural sweetener. Unripe bananas might not be palatable on their own, but blended into this smoothie they provide a great source of resistant starch fibre that helps support the gut. With some probiotic-rich kefir and raw honey added for good measure this is a great way to give your gut and your taste buds a morning boost.

serves 1

½ avocado

1 small–medium unripe banana

50ml kefir (dairy or coconut)

1 handful mung bean sprouts (optional)

2 tablespoons lucuma powder

1 teaspoon raw honey (substitute coconut blossom nectar for a vegan version)

toppings – a few suggestions

1–2 tablespoons lightly toasted coconut chips

1–2 tablespoons crushed almonds

1 tablespoon bee pollen (providing you don't have an allergy to bee products)

Place the avocado, banana, kefir, sprouts, lucuma and honey into a high-speed blender and blend to a creamy consistency.

Pour into a bowl and garnish with your choice of toppings.

raw coconut 'porridge'

Apples are one of the best sources of pectin, which provides a unique form of fibre for our beneficial gut bacteria. The humble apple forms the basis of this 'porridge' which, instead of using grains, has a mix of coconut and almonds – a welcome alternative for those who are coeliac or sensitive to grains. It's also an incredibly tasty mix and entirely satiating. The other key ingredient here is the Brazil nuts in the cream; they provide one of the highest sources of selenium, a powerful protective antioxidant for the gut. This is a marvellously moreish breakfast that all of the family will enjoy.

serves 2

1 large eating apple (green or red), cored and roughly chopped

75g activated almonds with skins (page 16)

20g coconut chips

1 teaspoon ground cinnamon

¼ teaspoon ground cardamom

1 pitted date

2 tablespoons cocoa nibs

Juice of ½ lemon

brazil nut cream

60g cashews, soaked for 2 hours

35g Brazil nuts, soaked for 4 hours

1 pitted date

Seeds from 1 vanilla pod

120ml filtered water

To make the Brazil nut cream, drain the nuts and rinse with filtered water. Place all of the ingredients into a high-speed blender and blend until smooth. Transfer to a glass or ceramic bowl and place in the fridge.

Place the apple, almonds and all the remaining porridge ingredients in a food processor and pulse until you have a sticky porridge-like consistency. Divide between two small bowls and serve with a generous tablespoon of the Brazil nut cream.

chicken bone broth

They say chicken soup is good for the soul – I say chicken broth is brilliant for the gut! That's because the bones contain nutrients such as amino acids, gelatin and collagen that help to support the intestinal barrier, so drinking this broth or using it in recipes at least two or three times a week is a great way to support a healthy gut. Bone broth also provides essential trace minerals such as calcium, magnesium and sulphur. Its awesome nutrition profile aside, bone broth is really tasty as a mid-morning drink and it gives depth of flavour to a simple soup such as my Spicy Parsnip Satay Soup (page 83).

Ask your local butcher or farmers' market for organic chicken carcasses or bones, including wings. It is crucial to use bones from organic free range chickens as these have a higher nutritional value.

makes 3–4 litres

3kg organic chicken carcasses, or 1 whole chicken carcass left over from a roast

Approx. 4 litres filtered water

3 tablespoons apple cider vinegar

1 large carrot

1 large celery stalk

1 large red or yellow onion

1 garlic clove

2 bay leaves

3 sprigs fresh thyme

1 tablespoon black peppercorns

Place the chicken pieces in a large cooking pot, add the water and vinegar and leave to stand for 20–30 minutes. The vinegar helps the nutrients in the bones become more readily available.

Thoroughly wash the carrot but don't peel it as there is a lot of nutrition in the skin; don't peel the onion or garlic, either. Roughly chop all of the vegetables and add to the pot along with the bay, thyme and peppercorns, making sure that the water covers the ingredients by a good 5cm.

Bring to a gentle boil then reduce the heat and simmer with a lid loosely covering the pot. Skim off and discard any foam that forms and check roughly every 20 minutes in the first couple of hours, skimming as necessary. When skimming you can also make sure the ingredients are fully covered with water and top up if needed. Simmer gently for 6 hours.

Remove the chicken pieces (you can save any meat from the bones to add to a salad or sandwich). Pour the liquid through a fine strainer into a large glass bowl; you can put the bowl into a sink of cold water or ice to speed up the cooling process. It is important to ensure that the broth is fully cooled before transferring into storage jars, otherwise you will have a breeding ground for less friendly microbes. Cover the jars and store in the fridge for up to 5 days or in the freezer for up to 1 month.

sauerkraut

OK, where do I start when it comes to the benefits of sauerkraut? Growing up with the stuff I guess I'm not new to it but it has rapidly gained popularity in recent years. Sauerkraut, or kraut as it's affectionately known, is fermented cabbage, which doesn't sound all that appealing, but trust me, once you start to eat this regularly you'll see how it can totally lift something simple like poached eggs on toast or what could be just another boring salad. Best of all it's one of the most abundant food sources of probiotics. Making it at home has many advantages as you know that it hasn't been pasteurised or heat-treated, in contrast to many of the shop-bought ones, plus there is something entirely satisfying about creating it yourself and connecting to your food. More to the point, it is easy to make and introduces trillions of beneficial bacteria to the gut.

makes about 400g (one large jar)

1 medium cabbage (you can use white or red or a mix of the two)

2 tablespoons mineral-rich salt

1 tablespoon caraway seeds

½ red chilli, deseeded and finely chopped (optional)

You will need: a large glass or ceramic bowl, a large wide jar with lid, some muslin cloth and a rubber band. Clean everything to give the beneficial bacteria the best chance to thrive. Clean your hands thoroughly, too.

Shred the cabbage into very thin strips and place in a large bowl. Add the salt and massage thoroughly to help release liquid from the cabbage until you get a mushy texture. This usually takes around 15–20 minutes, until you get a pool of liquid in the bottom of the bowl. Now add the caraway seeds and chilli, if using.

Place the cabbage in the jar and pack down as much as possible. Top with the liquid from the bowl so that it completely covers the cabbage (if there is not enough, then mix some filtered water with a little salt and add that).

Cover the jar with muslin cloth and a rubber band so the kraut can breathe. Press down every few hours, making sure the liquid covers the cabbage.

After 24 hours, cover the jar with a lid and keep it at room temperature for a further 3–4 days minimum. Your kraut should then be ready to eat, but you can leave it longer for extra flavour and fermentation. When it tastes the way you want it to, store in the fridge.

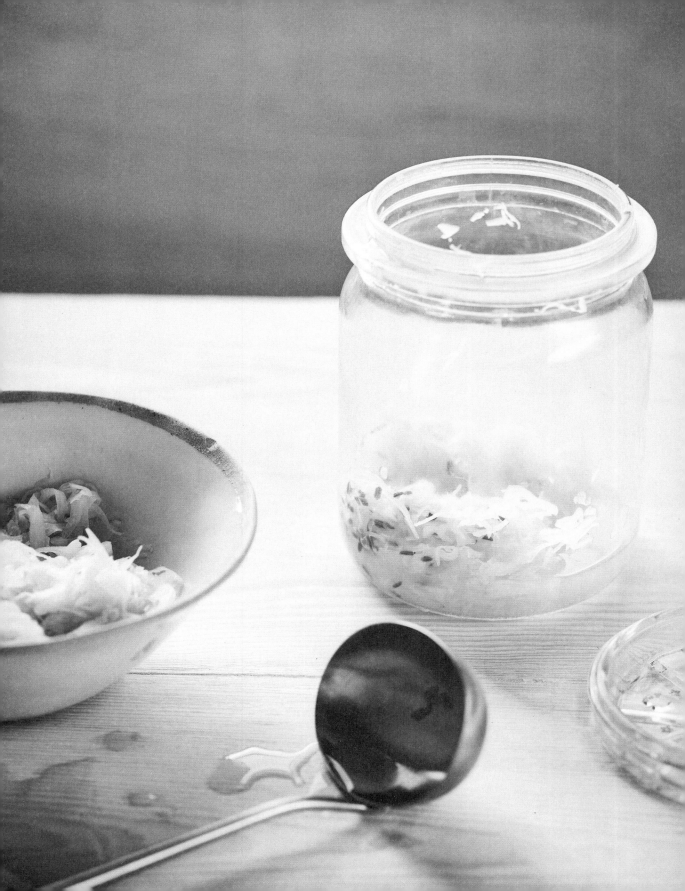

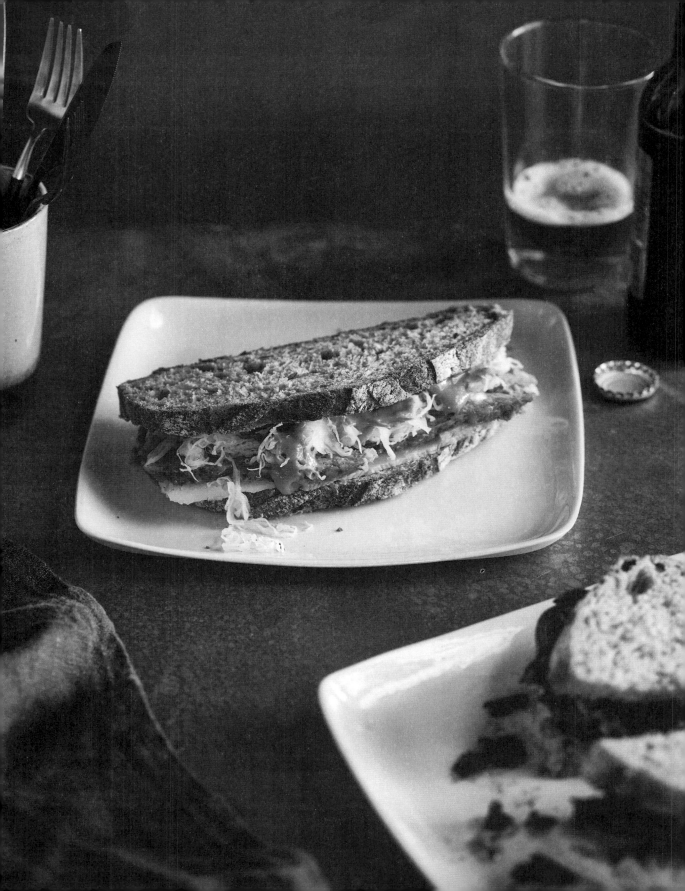

tempeh reuben on sourdough

After reminiscing about a magnificent Reuben I had in New York many years ago, I decided to recreate the delicious combination of flavours using my favourite fermented foods. This is a sandwich that is bursting full of natural probiotics and one that your gut is gonna love. Tempeh is made from fermented soya beans and sourdough is made by a process of fermentation. Add some probiotic-rich unpasteurised Manchego cheese and then a decent serving of sauerkraut, which is said to have more than a trillion bacteria in just one cup. This is off the spectrum when it comes to being gut friendly and it is big on flavour too!

serves 2

100g non-GMO tempeh
2 tablespoons tamari
½ teaspoon ground cumin
½ teaspoon paprika
4 slices sourdough
6–8 thin slices unpasteurised Manchego
45g sauerkraut (page 58), well drained

russian dressing

2 tablespoons cashew nut butter
2 tablespoons tomato paste
1 tablespoon apple cider vinegar
1 teaspoon onion powder
¼ teaspoon mustard powder
½ teaspoon smoked paprika
Pinch mineral-rich salt
3 tablespoons filtered water

Marinate the block of tempeh in the tamari, cumin and paprika for at least 30 minutes before you make your sandwich. Then cut the tempeh into thin slices, ready to assemble.

Put all the Russian dressing ingredients into a small bowl and whisk to combine, then put to one side.

To make the sandwich, start by laying out 2 slices of sourdough. Add a layer of the Manchego (which will help prevent a soggy sandwich bottom from the sauerkraut). Next add the tempeh and then the drained sauerkraut. Spread the other 2 sourdough slices with a generous tablespoon of the Russian dressing and flip over on top of the sauerkraut. Cut in half diagonally and enjoy.

tip

I think Manchego works best flavourwise, but you can use another unpasteurised cheese instead if you choose.

punchy potato salad

I know potato salad seems a tad retro, but cooked and cooled potatoes are one of the best sources of resistant starch, which helps bacteria to produce substances that support the health of the gut. When fully cooled, they contain a different type of starch from freshly cooked hot spuds, which don't have the same effect. This salad also contains probiotic badass gherkins that give an additional gut-friendly boost. This is brilliant on its own, or with some slices of unpasteurised halloumi mixed through. Whip it up for your summer barbecue parties as a delicious side salad. See my Happy Cow Burgers (page 180) for a great combo.

serves 2–3

225g baby new potatoes (approx. 10 potatoes)

1 tablespoon activated pumpkin seeds (page 16)

1 tablespoon activated sunflower seeds (page 16)

3 large unpasteurised gherkins

Generous handful of two fresh herbs (I like chervil and mint but you can use parsley instead of chervil; dill also works well)

Generous handful of rocket

1 tablespoon shelled hemp seeds

1 tablespoon tahini

Juice of ½ lemon

Generous pinch mineral-rich salt

Steam the potatoes the day before you want to eat this. Leave to cool then let them fully cool in the fridge overnight. If you haven't already done so, prepare your pumpkin and sunflower seeds.

To prepare the salad, finely slice the gherkins vertically, roughly chop the herbs and add to a large bowl, along with the potatoes. Add the rocket and the pumpkin, sunflower and hemp seeds.

In a small bowl, mix the tahini with the lemon juice and salt and a little filtered water to thin to a creamy consistency. Add this to the bowl with the salad and combine all together thoroughly.

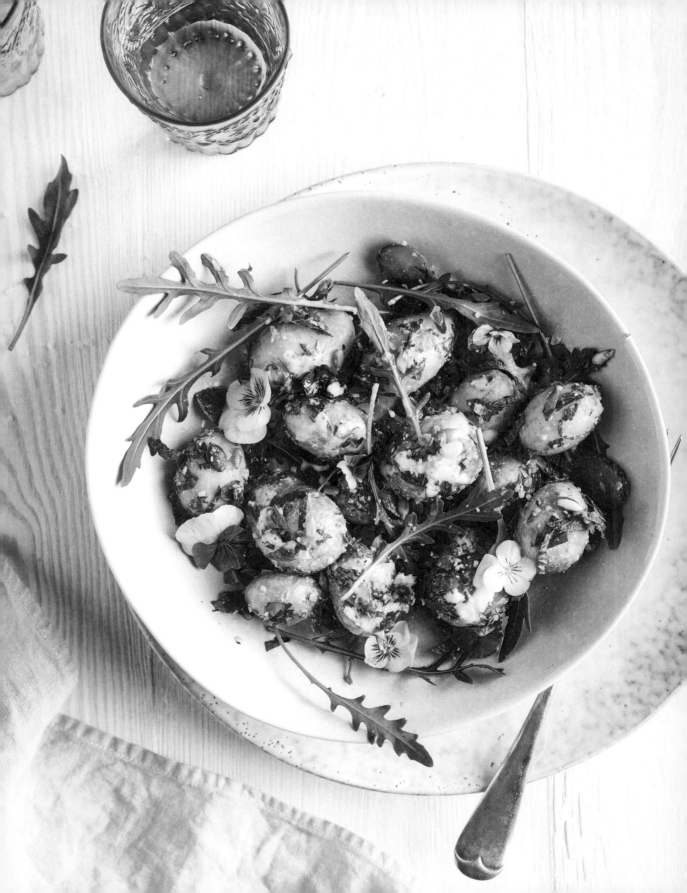

raw roots with fermented beets and labneh

This pretty salad needs a bit of prep in advance to ferment your beets and to make the labneh, but it's well worth it and a bit of a showstopper if you are entertaining. The beetroot and labneh not only taste incredible but also give so much back to your gut with their wealth of beneficial bacteria. And despite the time element they are really easy to make. I like this served alongside grilled wild salmon with some of my Super Seed Bread (page 157) on the side, but you can have it with just a few slices of the bread and a more generous portion if you prefer.

serves 2–4

fermented beets

4–5 small beetroots (if you like you can go for a mix of colours – pink, red, golden)

1 teaspoon coriander seeds

1 teaspoon fennel seeds

400ml filtered water (super important as this allows the bacteria to thrive, so make sure it is filtered or bottled)

1 tablespoon mineral-rich salt

labneh

¼ teaspoon mineral-rich salt

450g full fat organic sheep's milk yogurt

2 courgettes

8–10 radishes

2 tablespoons extra virgin olive oil, plus extra to drizzle

Generous squeeze fresh lemon juice

1 tablespoon tahini

2 tablespoons finely chopped fresh mint

2 tablespoons finely chopped fresh parsley

Generous pinch mineral-rich salt

You will need: two 500ml (or 1 pint) jars with lids, such as Mason jars; some muslin cloth.

To ferment your beets, first wash your jars thoroughly and make sure they are squeaky clean. Place ½ teaspoon of each of the seeds into each jar. Pour the water into a jug, add the salt and stir until fully dissolved. Slice the beets into 5mm slices and layer into the jars. Pour the salt water into the jars, making sure to cover the beets, leaving a gap of around 3cm at the top of each jar. Using a pestle or a wooden spoon, press down on the beets to make sure they are well covered. Add a touch more filtered water if needed. Put the lids on and leave to ferment at room temperature for 7–10 days. In the first week, remove the lids every day to release air; if your beets have started to rise out of the salt water, press down to re-submerge. After 7–10 days, screw the lid on tightly and store in the fridge for up to 1 month.

To make your labneh, stir the salt into the yogurt. Place the mixture into a large piece of muslin and tie the edges together to form a tight bundle. Hang this over a large bowl, suspending the bundle from a spoon, put in the fridge and leave to drain for 24 hours (or hang the bundle from a kitchen tap and leave to drain for 24 hours). After this the yogurt should be thick and dry, with its liquid in the bowl. Discard this liquid and transfer the labneh to a ceramic or glass container and store in the fridge. This will keep for up to 5 days.

To assemble the dish, slice the courgettes and radishes into thin rounds and lay on a large plate. Take 10–15 slices of the fermented beets and add to the plate. Mix the olive oil, lemon juice and tahini together in a small bowl. Then add 6–8 generous blobs of the labneh around the plate. Scatter with the herbs and drizzle with the dressing. Finish with a generous pinch of mineral-rich salt and another generous drizzle of olive oil.

tiger nut macaroons

Tiger nuts are not actually nuts; rather they are small tubers that contain resistant starch. This helps to 'feed' the beneficial bacteria in the gut to produce certain anti-inflammatory substances such as butyrate, which is vital for the health of the gut. Tiger nuts are surprisingly sweet and chewy but although they have been traditionally used in Spain to make a milk called horchata de chufa, many of us would not necessarily be familiar with them. Once you try them I promise you'll be hooked! These macaroons are excellent when you need a pick-me-up with a cuppa or as a dessert. Just don't scoff the lot in one go!

makes 16 macaroons

100g tiger nut powder
2 tablespoons cashew nut butter
45g desiccated coconut
40g coconut chips
Pinch mineral-rich salt

Place all the ingredients in a food processor and pulse until the coconut chips are broken down. Add 3 tablespoons of filtered water to help bind the mixture (you may need to add a little more; they should be moist but not too wet and sticky).

Remove from the processor and roll the mixture into 3cm balls. Flatten each ball on the base but leave a dome shape. Place in the fridge. They will keep for up to 1 week.

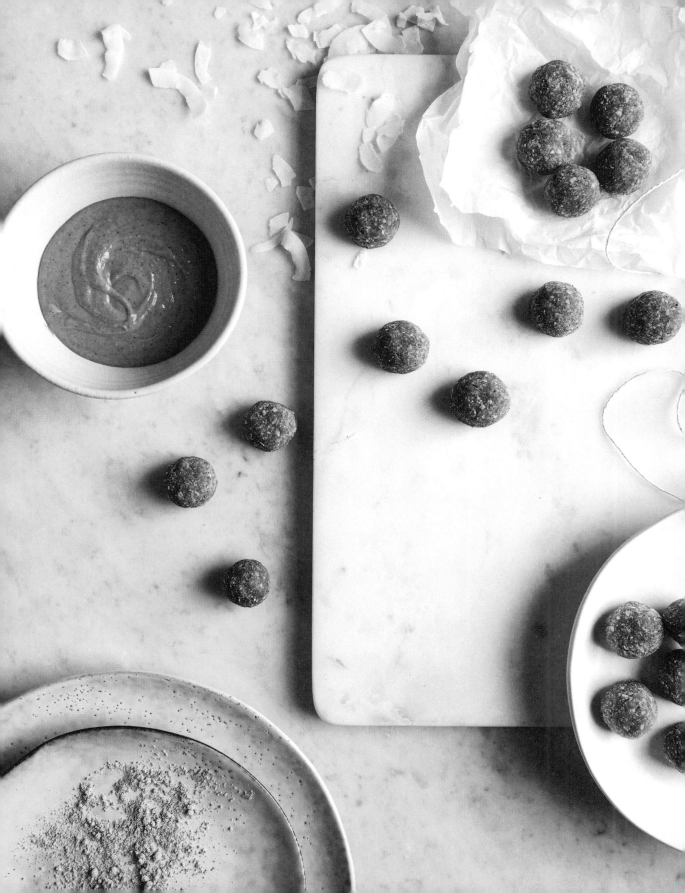

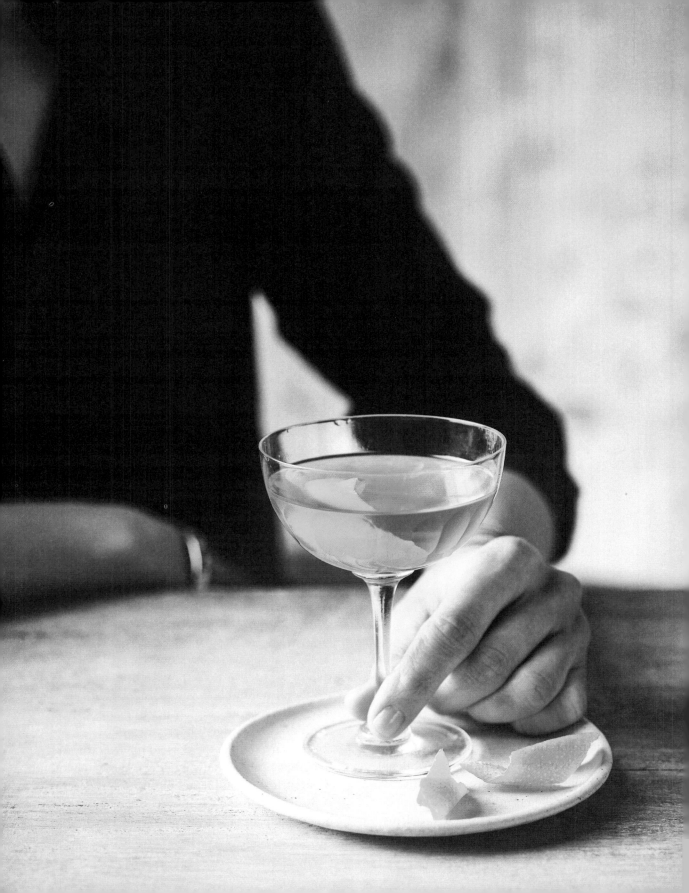

3

why it goes out of whack

I WOULD QUESTION *anyone* who says they have perfect digestion. In a world of refined and processed fast food, high consumption of sugars, copious amounts of artificial ingredients and chemical additives, we put our digestive systems under constant assault. To add insult to injury, we don't eat enough of the foods that help support a healthy gut and its trillions of resident bacteria. We also work ridiculously long hours and eat food rapidly, often on the go, putting our digestion under even more stress. It's no wonder the gut simply can't keep up.

As I'm sure many of you will have experienced at some point, the gut is very good at telling us when it is unhappy. Unfortunately, people often ignore or accept persistent digestive symptoms as 'the norm'. Over many years, however, these seemingly 'minor' problems

can accumulate and lead to some much more profound imbalances, so it's important to tune into your gut and ask, 'Are things really OK or have they shifted too far out of whack?'

Many digestive symptoms can be deemed idiopathic in their nature, which means they don't have one distinct cause. But there is always a reason (or reasons) why they occur, so the challenge is to work out what is at the root of the problem. That's what this chapter is about. I want to help you to understand how and why your gut may be struggling. With this knowledge, I hope you will be able to start 'joining the dots' to uncover the underlying cause of any niggling issues you may have, such as painful reflux or uncomfortable constipation. You may already be some way down that path of self-discovery but, equally, the next few pages can help you gain a more thorough understanding of factors that might be influencing your personal situation.

Whether you have a minor or more serious gut problem, this information is designed to help you figure out where your gut needs some attention and how best to support it. As you will have learnt in the previous chapters, healthy gut function depends on the balance of bacteria in the gut and the mechanical processes of digestion, underpinned by the right types of food to ensure it all runs smoothly. With that in mind, the recipes and foods in this chapter are there to use when the going gets tough – dishes like my Spicy Parsnip Satay Soup (page 83), which is a delicious and easily digestible hug for the gut, and my Carrot Cake 'Porridge' (page 82), which will help keep things moving along just how they should.

But to kick all of this off, we need to understand what constitutes a healthy movement and how much it can tell us about the health of our gut. Yep, we need to start talking poo.

the perfect poo

This heading might make you feel a tad uncomfortable but we can't dodge the issue because our daily 'movements' can tell us so much about what is happening in the gut – and it's time we took notice. I'm not suggesting you need to check your number twos obsessively, but noticing even subtle changes can give distinct clues to any imbalances in the gut and our health overall.

So let's start with the basics: what is poo (or a stool to use its official name)? Contrary to what many people believe, it is not simply the remnants of the food that we have eaten. It's much more interesting than that. Our stools are mostly made up of water (which is why constipation is often simply the result of dehydration), with the remainder being a combination of indigestible fibre, additional toxic substances that the body needs to get rid of (such as medications or cholesterol) and gut bacteria that have come to the end of their natural life. In fact, it is thought that just 1 gram of a stool contains more bacteria than there are stars in the universe.

Old blood cells are also transported out of the body via the stool, which accounts for its natural mid-brown colour. And colour is a very important marker indeed. If a yellow hue or a clay colour is evident, it can be indicative of some dysbiosis in the gut or liver and gall bladder issues. Bright red specks of colour can be caused by haemorrhoids while darker red or black stools are 'red flag symptoms' that should be checked out by your doctor. If you experience pain with your movements or bowels more generally then you should definitely seek further investigation.

When it comes to your movements, there are four key factors to monitor: regularity, consistency, efficiency and satisfaction.

Regularity means that once to twice a day spent on the bathroom throne is ideal. Any more or less than that means things are possibly not moving through the gut as they should be.

Consistency of our stool is also a good indicator of gut health. Ideally, it should look like a long soft log that is like an ice cream in texture. It should be fully formed, and should not have cracks or be too mushy. Hard little lumps and watery liquid would be the extremes of this. The Bristol Stool Chart is an excellent reference and illustrates perfectly how your poo should look (simply search for it online).

Efficiency Movements should be smooth, quick and pain free. Taking a book into the bathroom should not be a prerequisite!

Satisfaction When you have fully evacuated you should experience a sense of elimination 'euphoria' and finish with a smile on your face (not with the feeling that you'll be back on the throne in 10 minutes).

This is what we are ideally looking to achieve but it seems to be a rare experience for many people. Why is that and how can we achieve a more pleasant daily visit?

too slow to go

Constipation refers to infrequent and/or hard to pass movements and is said to affect 1 in 7 people on average. While the tendency is to focus on having a daily routine, which is the ideal, we need to be more aware of efficiency, and that means a quick, smooth and easy process.

Constipation can be due to many different causes but essentially it is the job of the nervous system to trigger an evacuation and if this is not working harmoniously with the other systems in the gut then the whole 'orchestra' can go out of sync. Many of us find that stressful situations and long-distance travel put bowel movements temporarily on hold. In the case of stress, the bowels tend to 'hold' as the body reverts to that knee-jerk, 'fight or flight' stress response. Travel-related constipation is often caused by the excitability of the trip and dehydration – airplanes are great at sucking moisture out of the body, and the bowel needs plenty of water for the simple act of elimination.

Ongoing constipation requires deeper analysis. Look into potential gut dysbiosis or undiagnosed thyroid issues, for example, with the help of your GP and a nutritional therapist. It is always best to try to avoid laxatives because long term use can disrupt the process of digestion and absorption. Tick the following three simple things off your list first if you need gentle help with nudging the process.

1. **Are you drinking enough fluid?** We need on average 2 litres per day and the bowels use a lot of this, so upping your water consumption can make things a little easier. We also need water to enable fibre to do its job properly, which leads nicely on to the next point.

2. **Are you eating enough fibre?** We need both insoluble and soluble forms, as they have different benefits in supporting the bowels. Luckily nature has made many fruit and veggies bountiful in both so try to eat a wide variety. Ground linseed or flaxseed can be particularly effective for 'slow movers'. And lightly stewed apples, which contain pectin, can also be a good bowel regulator, so have a look at my recipe on page 111. However, don't go overboard and suddenly start eating loads of fibre, particularly if your body is not used to it, as you may create other unpleasant symptoms. Your aim is to increase movements, not to have a brass band playing down there! Government guidelines say that our dietary fibre intake should be around 30g per day and if you are achieving your 5–10 portions of fruit and veg, with some sprouted or fermented grains as well as nuts and seeds, then you should meet your quota. If you experience more problems when

you increase your fibre intake, consider functional testing (see page 79), as you may have bacterial imbalances that need to be isolated and addressed first.

3. **Are you stressed?** Holding tension in your body means you are holding it in your gut, too. Try including practices such as yoga or meditation in your daily routine to help support relaxation. Fennel tea can act as a nice bowel relaxer so try steeping some seeds in hot water and see if that helps.

fast and furious

Urgency and/or diarrhoea are issues for many people. Sometimes there can be a specific reason for having to find a loo pretty swiftly: for example, severe bacterial or parasitic infections, often in the form of food or water poisoning; too much alcohol; laxative abuse; certain medications; or a flare-up of an intestinal disease such as Crohn's or ulcerative colitis. However, there can be reasons that are seemingly inexplicable and the phrase 'one man's food is another man's poison' often applies here. Undiagnosed food sensitivities or intolerances can be another reason for erratic, rapid bowel movements (we will look at what can cause these kinds of disruption and how to pinpoint them in Chapter 6). There may also be underlying imbalances in the microflora of the gut that are shifting the balance towards urgency.

If you suffer from constipation or diarrhoea (some people swing between the two) on a regular basis, and have ruled out other more serious gastrointestinal conditions, my Weed, Seed and Feed programme on page 46 can help to reduce or remove triggers and generally support the microbial landscape of the gut and hence better bowel habits.

digestive conditions

Now we turn our attention to some of the most common gut-related conditions. You may well have been diagnosed recently or could have suffered with one of these conditions for a long time. Alternatively, you might read through some of these and find the symptoms resonate with you, in which case you should seek further help from your GP to get a clear diagnosis, as well as seeking support from a registered dietician or nutritional professional. This section explains some of the underlying causes and suggests ways that may help you manage and alleviate certain symptoms. While I try to keep things as simple as possible, there are technical details that it is important to understand, so do stick with it through those sections.

reflux and gerd

A common tell-tale sign that all is not as it should be in your gut is reflux, which, in chronic cases, is better known as gastro-oesophageal reflux disease, or GERD. It is characterised by gastric juices (hydrochloric acid) from the stomach passing up into the oesophagus, causing a burning sensation in the throat and chest area. It can best be thought of as a signal failure between the stomach and the valve that separates it from the oesophagus. When the nervous systems of our gut and brain do not receive the correct information, reflux symptoms can arise. Situations that can throw out this connection include smoking and pregnancy, so reflux is often a complaint among smokers and pregnant women.

Medications that are commonly used to treat reflux include PPIs (proton pump inhibitors) or antacids. These can work as a short-term measure, but if the acid levels in the stomach are too low they can make a bad situation worse. This is actually more common than you may think. As I mentioned in Chapter 1, your stomach needs to be super acidic to break down food properly so that you can absorb all the nutrients. When you add these acid-lowering medications, the pH increases to around the same as vinegar, which has a negative impact on how efficiently we break down our food.

Stomach acid levels are also influenced by factors such as having enough zinc, hydration and the amount of stress we experience. If you have too much stress it can cause the body to increase or, conversely, inhibit the production of gastric juices and, for both high and low stomach acid, create similar symptoms. The simple baking soda test, right, will give you a rough idea of your levels and which way you need to go to swing the balance in the right direction.

You should also consider *how*, rather than what, you eat. The simple act of chewing properly and taking time over meals can have a marked impact both on reflux and bloating. Remember, food should be almost liquid in the mouth before swallowing, to avoid the stomach having to work that much harder to break it down. Around 15–20 minutes is really the minimum time to take over your meals. Time your next meal – you might be surprised at how quickly you gulp down your food.

Reflux can be caused by a bacterial infection in the stomach called *Helicobacter pylori*, which also causes ulcers and a burning sensation in the gut. It may also be due to an overgrowth of bacteria that have migrated into areas of the small intestine, a condition known as small intestinal bacterial overgrowth, or SIBO. In the latter case,

the baking soda test

If you have symptoms of reflux or heartburn, or other gut-related conditions such as irritable bowel syndrome (IBS), irritable bowel disease (IBD) or GERD, it may be a sign that your stomach acid levels are low. Try this simple home test to see how your level stacks up. It's not based on rigorous science but it can give some indication.

Complete the following test on three consecutive days so you get an average. You should do the test as soon as you wake up in the morning before you have eaten or drunk anything.

- Dilute ¼ teaspoon of baking soda in ½ cup of filtered cold water
- Drink the solution
- Time how long it takes you to burp.

If you have adequate amounts of stomach acid you should burp within 2 to 3 minutes. If it takes longer, it may be that you are not producing enough gastric juices. Remember to take your average time over the three days.

the gas produced by the bacteria can cause the small intestine to expand, putting pressure on the stomach and the oesophagus that results in a 'spilling over' of gastric juices. Furthermore, SIBO can lead to an inability to produce adequate digestive enzymes and poor absorption of nutrients, which can also slow down digestion and lead to a back-up of food and consequent reflux symptoms. (We will look at SIBO in more detail shortly.) *H. pylori* and SIBO can be detected via breath and stool tests respectively and then addressed accordingly.

tackling low stomach acidity

If you think you have low stomach acid levels there are some steps you can take to address this.

1. Try drinking apple cider vinegar immediately before each meal. Start with one tablespoon (diluted in a splash of filtered water if necessary). You should get a feeling of warmth in your stomach. If you don't experience that sensation, you can try up to 2 tablespoons or even 3 but note that a burning sensation means you have gone too far! The great thing about stomach acid is that it has a positive feedback mechanism so the body will respond by increasing your acid levels once you start to supplement.

2. If the apple cider vinegar isn't alleviating your symptoms, you could try a supplement that contains betaine hydrochloride (HCL). However, you should ideally work with a nutritional practitioner on this before going ahead (and should have ruled out high levels of acid production or you could make that burning sensation a whole lot worse).

3. My final tip is to eat a daily teaspoon of raw local or Manuka grade honey. Due to their antimicrobial properties, these specific types of honey can help to counteract bacterial overgrowth in the stomach. It is important to get the real stuff, rather than highly processed honey, which doesn't have the same benefits.

Alcohol consumption can also damage the acid-producing cells in the stomach, so be mindful of your alcohol intake if you suffer from reflux symptoms.

irritable bowel syndrome (IBS)

One of the most common digestive conditions is irritable bowel syndrome. Characteristic symptoms include abdominal pain and cramping (which may be relieved by a bowel movement), changes in the frequency or consistency of stools (such as constipation and/or diarrhoea), bloating, excessive gas, urgency and noticeable mucus in the stools. Other symptoms that can appear alongside these include nausea, fatigue, backache and bladder issues. Depression and anxiety are also very common in those with IBS.

Often categorised as a 'functional disorder', i.e. something with no known cause, IBS can be debilitating, painful and downright depressing. Thankfully there has been a move away from defining IBS in this way, which gives some hope that sufferers will no longer be fobbed off with 'there is nothing wrong', when clearly something is not working as it should. However, too many people are still given little or no explanation and few treatment options for a disorder that can be all-consuming. If you are suffering from IBS, you may need to do your own investigation. Obviously symptoms don't appear from nowhere so it's about tapping into your inner sleuth and uncovering some interesting correlations.

My advice? If you haven't already done so, start by cleaning up your diet. Bin the white, fried and dyed foods that offer little nutritional benefit and may be provoking symptoms. These are your typical junk foods and takeaways, such as pizza, crisps, chips, biscuits, ice creams and white breads. Our gut doesn't work well when we eat too much of this stuff. Instead eat lots of whole foods that don't come in a box or a bag, without labels or heating instructions. I'm talking foods in their most natural state. My Weed, Seed and Feed programme on page 46 is a good place to start.

Next you need to look at foods that may be triggering IBS symptoms. A food sensitivity or intolerance is different from an allergy, which can be life-threatening, but it can create unpleasant digestive symptoms nevertheless. (You can find out more about the distinction between the two in Chapter 6.) For those suffering with IBS, uncovering and avoiding trigger foods can certainly feel life-transforming. One common trigger food is gluten, a type of protein found in grain-based products such as bread, flour, biscuits and cakes. Recent studies show that 20 per cent of IBS patients with a suspected gluten sensitivity, but not coeliac disease (an allergy to gluten), tested positive for gluten antibodies, indicating a significant reaction to gluten when ingested. This means that gluten intolerance could well be a factor to consider as part of the bigger picture in IBS.

Other studies have suggested food groups such as certain types of dairy and histamine-releasing foods, including pork and beer, as possible digestive 'provokers'. However, when removing any foods that you suspect may be causing a problem, don't fall into the 'free from' trap and buy foods simply because they are labelled 'gluten-free' for example, as many of these include artificial ingredients that can be just as, if not more, disruptive to the gut. In particular, avoid processed soya products such as milks, creams, desserts and meat substitutes. Like other processed foods, these types of soya can also create symptoms in certain IBS individuals.

(For a more thorough discussion of elimination diets see Chapter 6.)

The FODMAP diet – an acronym that stands for fermentable oligosaccharides, disaccharides, monosaccharides and polyols – has been used in clinical settings with positive results for IBS patients. This diet essentially involves removing foods that contain these compounds. FODMAP foods are a collection of certain types of poorly absorbed sugars that are also present in wheat and dairy. Many people experience enormous relief on this diet but it's not really for the long term, as it means missing out on many of the foods that feed the beneficial bacteria in the gut such as apples, mushrooms and fermented foods. Garlic, onions and wheat-based foods seem to be the ones that provoke the most reaction, so you might try eliminating these first if you are suffering from IBS and see if that helps.

It might be a question of digging a little deeper (rather than just eliminating foods) and this is where a stool test (see page 79) can give a thorough picture of the microbiome. Potentially this could also give some clues as to the causes of your IBS. Hopefully, if your 'garden' simply needs a little bit of tending, the Weed, Seed and Feed programme will start to improve things.

irritable bowel disease (IBD)

Irritable bowel disease, or IBD, refers to a chronic inflammatory condition of the colon and small intestine. The term principally covers Crohn's disease and ulcerative colitis, which, unlike IBS, have visible symptoms, namely inflammation. This is usually diagnosed via a biopsy (performed as part of a colonoscopy) and the appearance of inflammatory markers in stool test results.

The location of the inflammation usually determines whether you are suffering from Crohn's disease or ulcerative colitis. Crohn's disease can affect anywhere in the digestive tract, right from the mouth to the anus, whereas ulcerative colitis tends to be more centred in the colon and rectum. While they are very different diseases, they produce similar symptoms – including bleeding, diarrhoea, vomiting, ulceration, extreme sharp pain and weight loss – and both are characterised by periods of flare-ups and remission. They also have another common denominator in that they are classed as autoimmune diseases, a term used to describe conditions in which the body attacks its own tissue – in these cases, the digestive system.

Most experts agree that a combination of genetics, environment, diet and a compromised gut microbiome can influence the onset of IBD. In fact, more and more research is alluding to the role that gut bacteria seem to play in the development of these diseases. Studies indicate that microbes can initiate, maintain and determine the onset of IBD. The theory is that an overgrowth of pathogenic bacteria creates alterations in the gut and the way that the immune system responds. This shift towards an imbalanced microbiome means that the lining of the gut may be damaged, a condition known as leaky gut, and this creates further immune system responses and inflammation. (We'll look at this subject in more detail in the next chapter.) Rebalancing the gut microflora

could therefore be considered an important part of the treatment of IBD.

Research in this area has led to the development of an intriguing and novel procedure – fecal microbiota transplantation. The aim of the treatment is to restore normal intestinal microbiota by transplanting microorganisms from a healthy person's stool into the gut of an IBD sufferer. The research is not extensive by any means but initial trials seem to have shown some positive results.

However, before you are tempted to go down that route, do not forget the marked influence of diet. This needs to be top of the agenda when treating IBD. Poor diet may have been one of the causes of bacterial imbalances in the first place, after all, and there are many studies to show how much improvement and management of irritable bowel disease can be achieved with relatively simple dietary adjustments. Eating foods that naturally support the health of the microbiome and removing potential dietary and lifestyle triggers, such as alcohol, smoking and gluten-containing foods, can help. Research shows that there is a correlation between gluten sensitivity and IBD. One study showed that by removing gluten from the diet, 65 per cent of participants reported an improvement in their symptoms and 38 per cent experienced fewer flare-ups in their condition. Using the FODMAP diet for a period of time can also be useful but it is important not to have too restrictive a diet, as that can result in nutritional deficiencies. For example, without adequate soluble fibre there is inadequate production of the anti-inflammatory short-chain fatty acids, such as butyrate, that we know to be crucial for gut health.

The starting point should be to support a healthy microbiome and work on bolstering the integrity of the gut, alongside an elimination diet. If you have been diagnosed with irritable bowel disease it is best to seek professional advice from a registered dietician or nutritional therapist, who will work with you and provide specific guided support.

small intestinal bacterial overgrowth (SIBO)

SIBO is a condition whereby microbes that should be staying in their home turf in the colon migrate to the small intestine, causing various problems. Bacteria should be present throughout the gastrointestinal tract but relatively few should hang out in the small intestine compared to the numbers in the colon, which should have the highest concentration. However, factors such as low gastric juice secretions, chronic stress, poor diet, gut infections, gastrointestinal diseases such as coeliac disease or Crohn's, or the overuse of antibiotics can cause pathogenic organisms to work their way up to the small intestine. Once this happens, the gut is in a state of dysbiosis and cannot function as it should. This affects the absorption of nutrients such as protein and fat, which can lead to deficiencies in amino acids and fat-soluble vitamins. These more disruptive bacteria can also 'snatch away' the B vitamins before our gut can absorb them and this can have a huge effect on energy processes among many other systems in the body.

The small intestine is also predominantly where our immune system is located. This is where the beneficial bacteria help crowd out more distruptive microorganisms and play a functional role in activating immune system tissue known as GALT (gut-associated lymphoid tissue). In the case of SIBO, these helpful microorganisms are outnumbered and depleted by less helpful bacteria and this can create damage to the mucosa, the cells that line the gut. This compromises the structure of the intestinal barrier, allowing food particles and inflammatory substances from bacteria out of the gut and into the bloodstream. This 'leaky gut' scenario can cause a cascade of immune reactions, such as food intolerances, and may increase the likelihood of autoimmune conditions, which often correlate with SIBO.

SIBO is often confused with IBS since the symptoms are very similar, and can be misdiagnosed. The typical constellation of digestive symptoms can include bloating, abdominal discomfort, gas, constipation and diarrhoea. While there isn't general consensus as to the best method of diagnosis, breath tests and cultures seem to be the most widely used and can certainly give some indication and basis for interpretation. SIBO is often treated using broad spectrum antibiotics, which in some cases are necessary but in others could have been a causal factor, so it's important to be discerning about how and when these are used. First get a diagnosis and then work with your GP, specialist and/or nutritional practitioner to find the best course of action for you.

Ultimately, you will need to work in conjunction with your health specialist to figure out the underlying cause or causes, based on the potential triggers, and look to address these, rather than blanket-bombing your body with antibiotics. The Weed, Seed and Feed programme on page 46 can help start the process, alongside the testing mentioned above. Don't forget the impact that lifestyle issues can have here. All the gut protocols in the world won't help you if you are under chronic levels of stress. Daily activities such as eating meals in an environment that allows you to 'rest and digest' is paramount, because often in cases of SIBO the 'inhale' approach to food has contributed to its development. Sit. Chew. Be present.

diverticulitis

Diverticular disease is a condition in which sac-like pouches called diverticula protrude from the lining of the colon. This can be asymptomatic but when these pouches become inflamed the result is diverticulitis. Symptoms can include pain, usually towards the left lower abdomen, nausea, constipation and sometimes diarrhoea. The condition usually appears later in life and although it is common there is fairly limited knowledge as to the cause and best treatment options.

Research has shown that sufferers of diverticulitis can also show imbalances in the gut microbiome and low grade inflammation of the gut, although it is thought that this inflammation could be triggered by dysbiosis in the gut in the first place – a bit of a catch-22 then! People with diverticulitis also often have altered colonic motility, which essentially means they have fewer bowel movements, and this could be another part of the picture to consider, as it might exacerbate bacterial imbalance. Other research has highlighted the fact that patients show disturbances in the gut serotonin system,

which is important since serotonin is a key player in keeping the gut moving. This links back to bacterial imbalances, which can negatively affect serotonin levels, since many beneficial bacteria are responsible for producing and managing serotonin in the body.

If you've been diagnosed with diverticulitis, or indeed diverticular disease, then rebalancing the gut, based on the results of some of the tests outlined in this chapter, is something you might want to consider. This should be done with a specialist in this area. Further to the serotonin point above, it's important to alleviate unnecessary stress as this can also contribute to flare-ups. Stress = inflammation, after all. So doing plenty of restorative activities, such as gentle yoga, walking and reading, should be part of helping to support your gut.

taking control

If your gut has been thrown off course, I hope this chapter has given you some food for thought that you can use to get it back on track. Whether that's embarking on the Weed, Seed and Feed programme as your starting point or working with a nutritional therapist and exploring stool analysis, there are many options that can help you take control of your gut health. Moreover, using some of the dedicated recipes in this chapter can help to gently nudge the gut in the right direction. Yes you may need to eliminate (albeit temporarily) some of those foods that could be causing issues for your gut, but try the recipes in this chapter, particularly my Chocolate Chia Fudgy Pancakes on page 81, and you'll understand why eating to get your gut working optimally can be decadent and delicious, too.

functional testing – why it's worth it

Finding the correct solution to an imbalance in your gut can be a long process that requires detective work in order to establish the cause. It's important, therefore, to understand the benefits of functional stool testing and how it can give diagnostic clues to the condition of your personal microbiome.

We know that the gut hosts trillions of microorganisms, some friendly, some not so friendly, and some that can create a lot of unpleasant side effects. With so many of these microbes in your gut, it can be near impossible to identify the specific ones that might be causing your symptoms or the processes that are out of alignment. Also, it isn't simply about obliterating the more pathogenic microbes but ensuring that there is an abundance of the probiotic bacteria to keep the gut functioning optimally. Stool testing is a great way to pinpoint where to target our ammunition, as well as where we need to boost our internal army of microbes. It also provides data on our digestive capabilities, such as the amount of digestive enzymes, and any raised inflammatory markers, both of which can help us form a wider picture of what's going on. This kind of comprehensive analysis allows for a more strategic and targeted approach to addressing potential imbalances and, while it is by no means a complete diagnosis, it can be a very important piece in the puzzle when it comes to supporting better gut health. You would need to run this kind of test through a nutritional therapist or similar specialist – see page 269 for more information on this.

However, the Weed, Seed and Feed programme on page 46 is a great place to start making fundamental changes and positive shifts in the gut. Using the elimination diet principles in Chapter 6 can also help you to uncover what works and what doesn't work for you. All of us are entirely unique, after all.

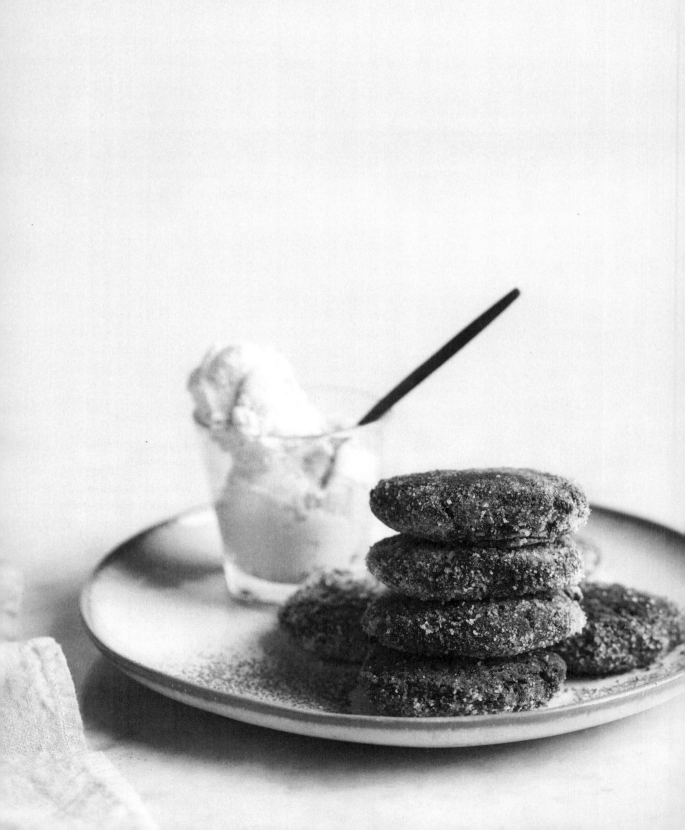

chocolate chia fudgy pancakes with coconut vanilla kefir

When it comes to breakfast, this recipe will have you springing out of bed in the morning. That could be down to the rich chocolate taste from the cacao powder – chocolate in its purest form. These pancakes are made from grain-free flours, so they are great for those who are gluten- or grain-sensitive. They also use chia seeds – rather than eggs – to bind, so they work for vegans, too. All that aside, these pancakes are deliciously gooey and perfectly satiating. It is best to make the coconut kefir in advance so it can chill and set, but if you haven't got time then you can serve the pancakes with unsweetened coconut yogurt instead.

serves 2 (makes 6–8 small pancakes)

pancakes

2 tablespoons chia seeds

120ml warm filtered water

50g coconut flour, plus 2 tablespoons for dusting

30g chestnut flour

4 tablespoons cacao powder, plus a little extra to serve (optional)

½ teaspoon bicarbonate of soda

200ml unsweetened cashew (or almond) milk

3–4 drops vanilla extract or seeds from 1 vanilla pod

2 teaspoons apple cider vinegar

2 teaspoons coconut oil for frying

coconut vanilla kefir

125g cashews, soaked for 2 hours, then drained and rinsed with filtered water

40g desiccated coconut

150ml kefir (dairy or coconut)

Seeds from 1 vanilla pod

Pinch mineral-rich salt

First make the coconut vanilla kefir: it needs at least 1 hour to chill and set, or you can make it in advance as it will last in the fridge for up to 3–4 days. Put all of the ingredients into a high-speed blender and blend until smooth. You will need to use the tamper to push down the ingredients, or stop and scrape a few times. Transfer to a sealable glass or ceramic container and place in the fridge for at least 1 hour.

To make the pancakes, mix the chia seeds and water in a bowl and leave for around 5 minutes until sticky.

Sift the flours, cacao powder and bicarbonate of soda into the bowl with the chia mix. Add the milk, vanilla and vinegar and stir to combine well. The mixture should be very thick and dough-like; you may need to add a bit more coconut flour so you can roll the mixture into one big ball without it sticking to your hands – if so, add it gradually.

Divide the dough into six to eight smaller balls and flatten into pancakes around 1cm thick. Dust with a little extra coconut flour on both sides, to stop them sticking to the pan.

Heat the coconut oil in a non-stick shallow pan over a low heat. Add the pancakes (you might need to cook them in two batches). Cook for 2–3 minutes, then flip and cook for a further 2–3 minutes. Serve on a plate, lightly dusted with cacao powder if you wish, alongside the coconut vanilla kefir cream or coconut yogurt.

carrot cake 'porridge'

This is a porridge with a difference, since it is based on ground flaxseed, which is great for keeping the gut moving and feeds our beneficial bacteria, too. Microbes also love feasting off the fibre in carrots, and along with some potent anti-inflammatory spices this breakfast makes a wonderful morning gut soother. Maca powder, which comes from a Peruvian root vegetable and is naturally sweet, helps to manage stress responses in the body, so you get off to a much calmer start.

makes 1 generous serving

1 carrot, peeled and cut into chunks

3 tablespoons ground flaxseed

2 tablespoons desiccated coconut

2 teaspoons maca powder

2 pitted dates

1 teaspoon raw honey

25g activated walnuts (page 16)

1 teaspoon ground turmeric

1 teaspoon ground cinnamon

¼ teaspoon ground ginger

Pinch nutmeg

Pinch black pepper

Place the carrot chunks in a food processor and pulse until you have finer pieces. Add all of the other ingredients and pulse until the chunks stick together. You may want to add a touch of filtered water.

Serve in a bowl, with warm almond milk and/or a generous tablespoon of coconut yogurt.

tip

Grinding your flaxseed from whole, fresh seeds is ideal to obtain maximum benefits. Always store your flaxseed in the fridge as it can go rancid quite quickly. Check out my shopping guide for a source of sprouted flaxseed.

spicy parsnip satay soup

Parsnips, like other root veg, are an excellent source of fibre that in turn helps our gut microbes to produce anti-inflammatory substances. The onion and garlic are prebiotic foods that also help support our microbial army. This soup is based on organic chicken bone broth, which is packed with amino acids that help to maintain a healthy gut lining. And the peanut butter, coconut and spices create a sweet satay flavour that is nourishing not just for the digestion but also for the soul. Serve with a generous slice of buttered sourdough. Yum.

serves 2

2 small–medium parsnips, peeled and cut into small chunks

1 red onion, peeled and quartered

2 garlic cloves, peeled

1 tablespoon unsweetened peanut butter

2 tablespoons desiccated coconut

8 dried lime leaves

Pinch chilli powder or flakes

2 teaspoons ground turmeric

2 teaspoons ground galangal

2 teaspoons ground cumin

½ teaspoon mineral-rich salt

Pinch black pepper

500ml organic Chicken Bone Broth (page 57)

Preheat the oven to 200°C/Gas 6. Line a baking tray with baking parchment.

Place the parsnips, onion and garlic on the baking tray and roast for about 20 minutes until tender.

Put the roasted vegetables into a high-speed blender and add all the remaining ingredients. Blitz until smooth and creamy.

Pour into a saucepan and heat gently for about 5 minutes, then divide between two bowls and serve.

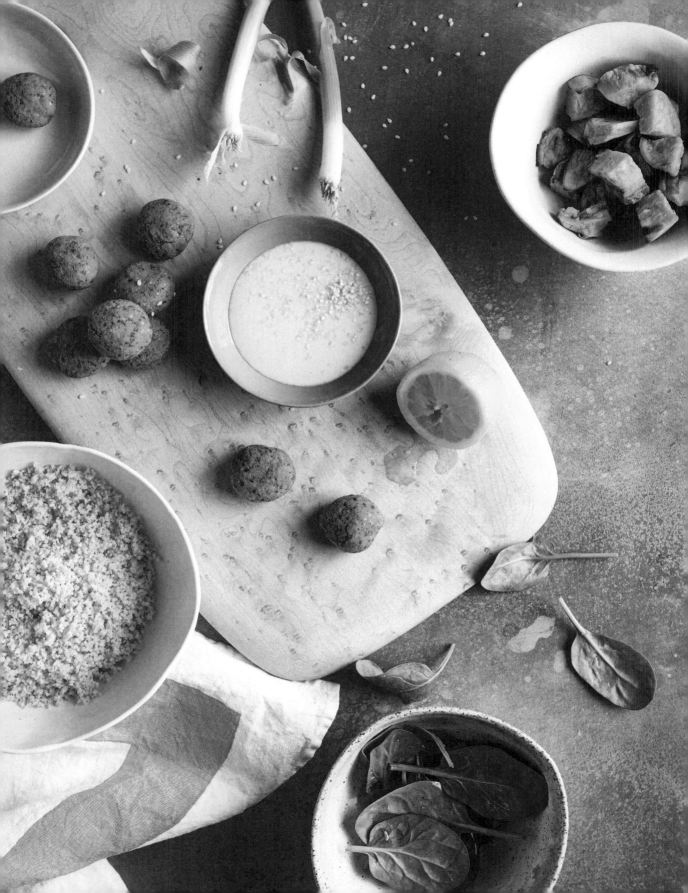

sweet potato falafel with parsnip 'couscous'

Sweet potato makes banging falafel and provides some really great fibre for the gut. It is also one of the highest sources of the antioxidant beta-carotene, which helps protect against cellular wear and tear. Making 'couscous' out of parsnips is an excellent alternative to the wheat-based version and can be a bit easier on digestion if you have a sensitive gut. This is served with a simple tahini dressing and a baby leaf spinach salad on the side. Why not double the quantities and have some for lunch the next day?

serves 2 (makes 10 falafel)

falafel

1 sweet potato, peeled and cut into chunks

2 spring onions, roughly chopped

1 tablespoon roughly chopped fresh coriander leaves

2 teaspoons ground cumin

1 teaspoon smoked paprika

½ teaspoon finely chopped fresh chilli (or a sprinkle of chipotle chilli)

½ teaspoon garlic powder (or 1 fresh garlic clove, crushed)

1 tablespoon fresh lemon juice

1 teaspoon almond nut butter

1 tablespoon sesame seeds

1 tablespoon coconut flour

Generous pinch mineral-rich salt

1 teaspoon ghee or organic butter for frying (use coconut oil for a vegan version)

tahini dressing

2 tablespoons tahini

Juice of 1 lemon

parsnip 'couscous'

2 parsnips, peeled and cut into small chunks

1 teaspoon ground cumin

Pinch mineral-rich salt and black pepper

1 teaspoon ghee or organic butter for frying (use coconut oil for a vegan version)

method overleaf

sweet potato falafel with parsnip 'couscous' method

Preheat the oven to 220°C/Gas 7. Line a baking tray with baking parchment, add the sweet potato chunks and roast for 25 minutes until tender.

While the sweet potato is cooking, prepare the other falafel ingredients and then add them all, except the ghee or butter, to a food processor.

You can also prepare the tahini dressing at this stage – simply mix the tahini and lemon juice and put to one side.

Once the sweet potato is tender, add it to the food processor. Pulse to get a smooth consistency, which will take about 5 minutes. You may need to stop and scrape the sides a couple of times.

Remove the mixture from the processor and, using 1 tablespoon per falafel, roll into small balls. Place to one side until ready to cook.

Wash the food processor. Add the parsnip chunks to the processor and pulse until you get a couscous-like texture. Add the cumin and seasoning and give a quick final pulse. In a saucepan on a low heat, melt the ghee, butter or oil and cook the couscous for 5 minutes. Divide between two plates.

To cook the falafel, melt the ghee, butter or oil in a frying pan and fry for 2–3 minutes, turning regularly to cook evenly. Serve on the couscous and drizzle with the tahini dressing.

pine nut parmesan

This is a fab recipe that you can sprinkle over everything from eggs in the morning to soup, veggies and salads. It's a great vegan alternative to cheese, perks up any dish immediately and is really handy to have in the fridge.

makes 1 small bowl

125g activated pine nuts (page 16)
90g flaked almonds
6 tablespoons (20g) nutritional yeast flakes
1 tablespoon fresh lemon juice
½ teaspoon mineral-rich salt

Place all the ingredients in a food processor and pulse for about 1 minute until you get a fluffy texture. Transfer to a sealable glass or ceramic container and store in the fridge for up to 1 month.

coconut blt

I first came across 'raw bacon' on an inspiring trip to LA many years ago: it really is the place for trailblazing vegan cuisine. Now don't get me wrong, I love a bit of organic free range bacon, but this alternative is great for a couple of reasons. Firstly, it is always good to extend our 'meat free' repertoire; and secondly, because you can make more than is needed for one sandwich, it makes a welcome crunchy topping for a salad or a tasty snack. Using avocado as a base for a vegan mayo gives another delicious layer of flavour and it is brim-full of beneficial fats and gut-supportive nutrients. This has me saying 'nom nom' every time I make it!

serves 2 (with extra mayo)

4 slices sourdough

Handful lettuce, either whole leaves if small or roughly chopped

2 tomatoes, cut into thin slices

coconut 'bacon'

40g coconut chips

2 teaspoons smoked paprika

2 teaspoons ground cumin

2 generous pinches mineral-rich salt

6 tablespoons (90ml) coconut aminos (or use tamari but reduce to 4 tablespoons)

avocado mayo

½ avocado

30g sunflower seeds, soaked for at least 2 hours, drained and rinsed with filtered water

2 tablespoons fresh lemon juice

1 tablespoon apple cider vinegar

½ teaspoon yellow mustard powder

2 teaspoons filtered water

50ml extra virgin olive oil

Generous pinch mineral-rich salt

Preheat the oven to 150°C/Gas 2.

To make the coconut bacon, place the coconut chips in a bowl and thoroughly coat with the paprika, cumin, salt and coconut aminos. Spread on a baking tray and bake for 15–20 minutes, stirring it around a few times so it becomes evenly crisp. Remove from the oven and leave to cool on the tray. Once cooled, store the 'bacon' in a sealable glass or ceramic container and keep in the fridge for up to 7 days.

To make the avocado mayo, put all of the ingredients in a high-speed blender and blend on the highest setting until thick and smooth; you may need to add a touch more filtered water.

To assemble the sandwich, start with a slice of sourdough, add a generous tablespoon of the mayo and spread to coat the bread. Then add the lettuce and a layer of tomato slices. Add a generous handful of the coconut bacon. Top with the other slice of sourdough. Cut in half and enjoy.

crab cakes with cashew dijonnaise

These cakes are a great option for a light lunch and can be cooked in advance to pack into a lunchbox. My take on a dijonnaise sauce doesn't have any of the hidden ingredients you might find in shop-bought versions and it goes perfectly with crab cakes. Serve them with a leafy green salad that includes half a sliced avocado and a sprinkling of pumpkin seeds. They also go really well with my Celeriac and Courgette Fries (page 177).

serves 2 (3 cakes each)

1 organic free range egg
100g white crab meat
1 spring onion, finely sliced
¼ teaspoon garlic powder
1 tablespoon unsweetened coconut yogurt
1 tablespoon chopped fresh dill, plus extra to garnish
1 tablespoon fresh lemon juice
2 pinches mineral-rich salt
3 tablespoons coconut flour, plus 2 tablespoons for dusting
2 teaspoons coconut oil

cashew dijonnaise

1 tablespoon cashew nut butter
¼ teaspoon mustard powder
1 teaspoon apple cider vinegar
1 teaspoon onion powder

To make the crab cakes, whisk the egg in a bowl and then add the rest of the ingredients, except the coconut oil. Mix to combine thoroughly. Place in the fridge for 10 minutes.

While the crab mixture is chilling, place the cashew dijonnaise ingredients in a small bowl and mix to a creamy, fairly thick consistency; add 1–2 tablespoons of filtered water to thin. Place to one side.

To prepare the crab cakes, take 1 tablespoon of the mixture, roll into a small ball and flatten to around 1cm thick. Dust on both sides with a little coconut flour and place to one side while you prepare the remaining cakes.

To cook the crab cakes, heat a frying pan on a low heat, add the coconut oil, then lightly fry the cakes for 3 minutes on each side. Serve with a generous tablespoon of the cashew dijonnaise and sprinkle with dill.

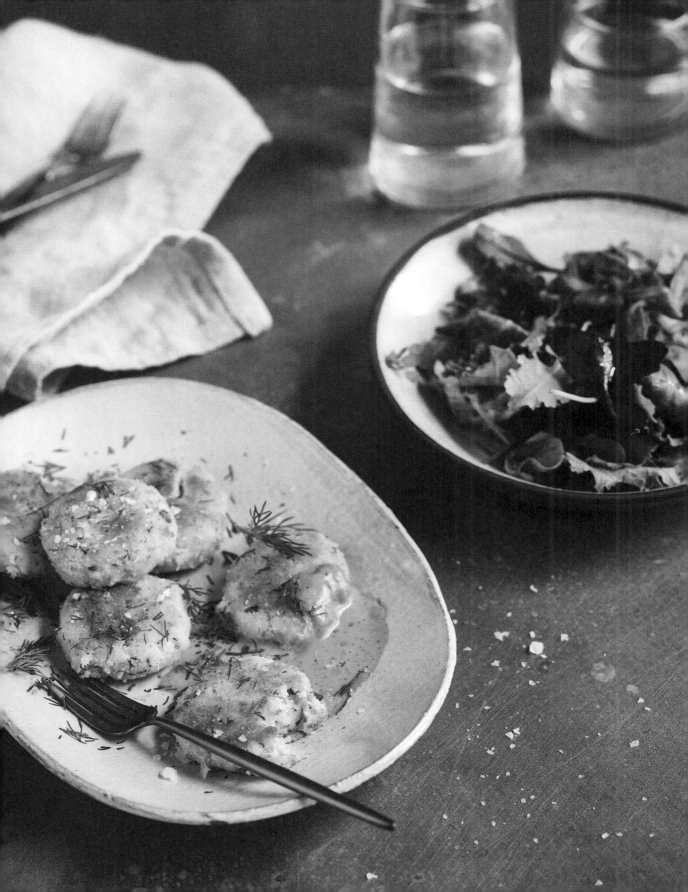

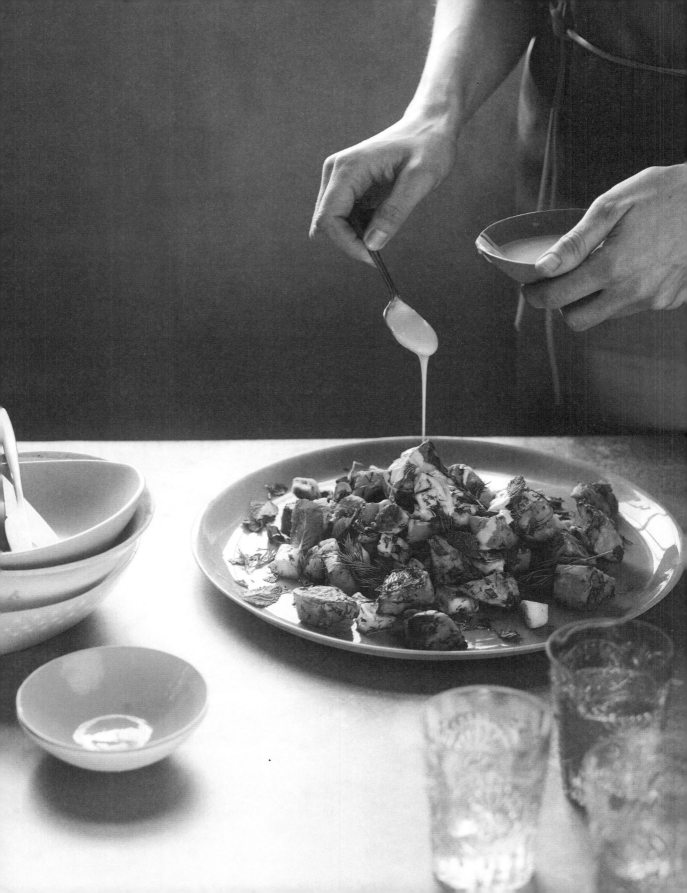

your natural armour

IN THIS CHAPTER we'll look at your natural armour – the immune system. Your gut and microbiome play a huge role in keeping your immune system firing on all cylinders, so I'll explain how our 'troops' in the gut are managed and primed, ready for action, and what happens when too many invaders take over. I'll look into the ramifications that a compromised microbiome has for the immune system, which can include autoimmune diseases and the somewhat controversial intestinal permeability, or 'leaky gut', and guide you through how to help restore gut equilibrium.

There are some exceptional foods that can help to boost immunity, including raw honey, kefir and mushrooms, so as well as exploring why they are ammunition for our internal gut army, I've included them in recipes such as my comforting Cauli 'Polenta' with Shimeji and Hazelnuts (page 104), the spectacular Tirami-shroom dessert (page 113) and the wonderfully nourishing Stewed Cinnamon Apples with Raw Honey Kefir Cream (page 111). One mouthful of any of these and your taste buds will be ready for action too!

manning the enemy lines

The gut is our largest immune organ, accounting for approximately 80 per cent of all immune cells and cellular hard wiring in the body. While we have other physical and mucosal barriers working to protect us from infection, including the skin and enzymes in tears and saliva, most of our body's natural armour is located within the lining of the gut.

Comprising just a single layer of cells that separates the rest of the body from substances entering from the outside world, high vigilance is needed along this vulnerable barrier. Policing what can and cannot get through is largely the responsibility of the gut's immune system, known as GALT (gut-associated lymphoid tissue). The gut wall is protected by secretions from GALT, the key one being SIgA (Secretory Immunoglobulin A), which can neutralise unwelcome invaders. Should these uninvited substances sneak past the SIgA surveillance and enter the mucosal layer, GALT calls up its second layer of defence – an army of immune cells that target and destroy the offending invader.

GALT relies on intricate 'conversations' between microbes in the gut and our immune cells to distinguish friend from foe and to react appropriately. After all, it has to perform the highly complex task of acting as a barrier to unwanted substances, such as toxins and pathogens, while also understanding when to allow through the nutrients that the body needs.

pac men, terminators and microbial bosses

So how do the immune cells in the gut recognise a foe? The answer lies in antigens, the small marker molecules attached to the surfaces of pathogens (a pathogen is basically any agent that can cause disease). The immune system recognises the antigen as harmful and obliterates the pathogen that is trying to gate-crash the party. This process happens regardless of whether or not the immune system has previously come into contact with the particular pathogen. However, each time certain cells of the immune system (B cells, a type of white blood cell) are exposed to a new, unfamiliar antigen they produce an antibody to it so it can be disposed of before it can infect other cells. Here's where it gets clever – the immune system 'memorises' its reaction so that it can be ready with a more targeted, efficient response when the body next comes into contact with the same pathogen. (This has important connotations for how we react to certain foods, as we'll see later.)

Like any strong army, this needs the right back-up, which is where macrophages, another type of white blood cell, come in. Like little pac men, they gobble up cellular debris, foreign substances, bacteria and any other defunct cells in a process called phagocytosis. Macrophages, like B cells, are under the guidance of what are called T helper cells, which alert the rest of the immune system to potential threats by secreting cytokines (hormonal messengers in the immune system) that stimulate the appropriate immune response. Gathering the rest of the troops, they switch on B cells, rally macrophages and also activate 'killer' T cells, or what I like to call terminators, to target infected cells. Within the T helper cell ranks are two main sub-types: Th1 cells, which are directed towards infections by viruses and certain bacteria and could be described as the first line of defence against pathogens; and Th2 cells, which are associated with bacteria and allergens and stimulate the production of antibodies in response to pathogens found in blood or other bodily fluids. Crucially, for the immune system to operate on an even keel, there needs to be a balance between the two.

Overseeing and coordinating these T helper cells are regulatory T cells, or T-regs. These are important since we don't want an immune system that overreacts and kills everything it comes into contact with, including our own cells. Yes we need a vigilant watch but we also want one that knows when to stand down. T-regs manage this anti-inflammatory response and counterbalance the other more 'confrontational' immune cells.

But who is in charge of this entire immune operation? It turns out that the bosses are our gut microbes. Not only do these microbes signal to the immune system that they are welcome guests but recent evidence shows that they instruct the T-regs to stay calm via markers on their surfaces, and by producing chemicals that pacify rather than provoke the immune system. Gut microbes also provide a 'boot camp' for the immune system, 'educating' it to differentiate between beneficial and more pathogenic microbes, as well as tissue that is self and non-self. The role of the gut microbiome is therefore of paramount importance for immune system regulation.

Given this military-like operation, it's much easier to understand why imbalances in the gut can create a cascade of catastrophic results for the immune system, and why nourishing our microbiome leads to a sturdier and wiser immune army.

living in an immune-challenged world

Our immune systems appear to be facing unprecedented assault, as demonstrated by the rising number of people suffering from autoimmune diseases. Evidence suggests that in Westernised societies the prevalence of these diseases has increased dramatically over the past 30 years, and the numbers continue to rise. There are over 80 recognised autoimmune disorders, some of which you wouldn't necessarily realise come under that umbrella term. These include Hashimoto's thyroiditis, Type I diabetes, fibromyalgia, psoriasis and rheumatoid arthritis, plus many more, each with its own unique symptoms. And while these disorders differ in their expression, their basic cause is the same: the system that should suppress defective immune cells instead allows them to go on an inflammatory and self-destructive rampage and destroy healthy body tissue – self attacks self in other words. This damage is usually directed at a specific system or area of the body. So, for instance, in Crohn's disease the intestinal tract is affected, whereas multiple sclerosis affects the central nervous system.

Autoimmune diseases don't happen overnight. On the contrary, 'unexplained' symptoms may go on for many years and include headaches, anxiety, brain fog, dry or flaking skin, acne, allergies, joint stiffness, fatigue and gastrointestinal symptoms, to name but a few. So if you have some of these symptoms for an extended period, don't ignore them.

so what is going wrong?

There are many theories as to the causes of autoimmune diseases. Previously it was thought that they were almost entirely due to genetic predisposition, but the influence of our environment, or at least a combination of the two, is now also recognised as crucial. Environmental factors include things such as the food we eat, toxins in our environment and of course stress. And all of these factors affect the microbes in the gut, those sergeant majors of the entire operation. If there are not enough of these 'elite officers' to train the immune cells, it compromises the system and makes it susceptible to errors. Essentially the way is left open for untrained, rogue immune cells to wreak havoc in the immune system.

So what might be influencing these cells to go so far wrong? Research has linked certain microorganisms to specific autoimmune diseases and it is thought that these infections may trigger the onset of autoimmunity, especially in those with a genetic predisposition. Specifics aside, if there is gut dysbiosis, from overgrowth of pathogenic microorganisms and/or not enough beneficial bacteria, then this will impact on the functioning of the immune system.

why we all need a vigilant army

It has been suggested that in some conditions pathogenic microorganisms can also play a part in compromising the integrity of the gut wall, which is referred to as intestinal permeability or leaky gut. A more permeable intestinal barrier can allow pathogens, and the toxins in their cell membranes, to enter the bloodstream, which can elicit an instant inflammatory immune response, since these bacteria should be contained in the gut. But here's where the problem increases, because it has also been suggested that the same pattern can occur when food molecules escape from the gut and into the bloodstream. This is believed to be caused by repeated exposure to the same foreign food invader, which elicit the efficient 'memorised' response from the B cells of the immune system (see page 92). This can become compounded,

since some of these roaming bacteria, and potentially food molecules, can mimic some of our own tissue, with the result that the immune system becomes confused as to what it should destroy and what is acceptable. This has been termed molecular mimicry. Now that might sound like a trick a wizard might perform but you could think of it simply as a case of mistaken identity. The theory behind this is that foreign antigens such as bacteria or a virus can share similar, even identical, amino acid sequences or surface structure to our own tissue so, rather than reserving its best killer antibodies for these invaders, the immune system also attacks 'look-a-like', healthy tissue.

Certain types of bacteria and viruses can have this effect. The Epstein-Barr virus, for example, which is associated with glandular fever and typically causes chronic fatigue, seems to mimic the surface structures of tissue in the central nervous system. This means that while the immune system is trying to rid the body of this virus it may also damage vital nerve tissue. This type of copy-cat behaviour seemingly doesn't just happen as a reaction to bacteria and viruses. There are studies to indicate that the same process can occur with certain foods. This research suggests that foods that have the same antigen-sequencing structure as our own tissues can result in the production of antibodies not solely to those foods but, in the same pattern described above, also to healthy tissue. This response was found to be particularly relevant to some of the most commonly eaten foods, such as milk and wheat, and it has been suggested that such cross-reactivity might be one of the factors in the development of autoimmune diseases, as our own tissues continually get caught in the firing line.

This is why it's so important to have gut barriers that are nice and tight. If bacteria and foodstuffs aren't escaping into areas where they attract the attention of the immune system, it can target its resources to deal more effectively with genuine threats from external sources.

if you have an autoimmune disease

If you have been diagnosed with an autoimmune disease, depending on the type and severity, there are some things you can do to help support your gut and, as such, your immune system. Removing potential triggers could be a good place to start and can help create a much calmer situation all round. It could be worth considering eliminating wheat grains and conventional cow dairy products as these typically tend to be the most problematic, and also circumvents the 'mistaken-identity' scenario linked to these foods, as described earlier. If you go down this route, it is best to work with a trained professional to make sure you don't miss out on crucial nutrients. Ruling things out carte blanche isn't smart or necessary for everyone.

Most importantly add key nutrients to your diet, including the gut-healing amino acids that are found in foods like bone broth, and healthy fats, such as coconut oil and coconut milk. Omega 3 fatty acids also provide anti-inflammatory nutrients that are a crucial part of this process, so think oily fish, flax and chia seeds as well as the spice turmeric, which studies show helps to manage inflammatory responses in the body. Incorporating these foods into your diet can help to support the gut and the immune system.

should i have a food intolerance test?

You may be tempted to invest in a food intolerance test (usually called an IgG test) but frankly I often find these to be a bit of a waste of money. Yes they give a complete analysis of food reactivity but they also throw up a lot of false negatives. If you have a leaky gut (which we'll look at in more detail shortly), then you may find that the test flags up a lot more foods than those that are actually causing a problem. The reason for this is that they are potentially leaking out of the gut and eliciting an immune response, so it's not the food per se that's the problem but more that the lining of the gut is compromised. I recommend you work on healing the gut first and foremost, alongside dietary interventions, before going down that road. See Chapter 6 for more on food intolerance.

It's also a good idea to bolster those bossy beneficial bacteria in the gut, so that the rest of the 'troops' know what they are doing. Eating plenty of probiotic foods, such as unpasteurised sauerkraut, kefir, kimchi and miso, will provide natural sources but also consider taking a probiotic supplement. Check out the shopping guide (page 266) for recommendations.

Anyone with an autoimmune disorder would be well advised to have a blood test to determine their vitamin D levels, as a deficiency of this vital nutrient is common in sufferers, and you may need to supplement. Alternatively, you could

the immune honey pot

Real 'raw' honey is an immune powerhouse. In its raw state, honey contains thousands of beneficial enzymes, many essential amino acids and countless vitamins and minerals. It also contains unique phytonutrients, namely bee pollen and propolis, which help to modulate the immune system and counteract seasonal allergies. This is because raw honey contains small amounts of pollen that gently stimulate and strengthen the immune system, which is the reason why you should source honey that is local to your environment, as this will expose you to pollen from your immediate surroundings.

It also supports a healthy balance of bacteria in the gut since it promotes the growth of beneficial microorganisms and helps to crowd out those that are more disruptive.

Raw honey in its purest form will be on the cloudy side because it is taken directly from the honeycombs with minimal intervention. It should not be confused with the refined, heat-treated syrupy junk that you get in most supermarkets. That stuff is a far cry from its original elixir form.

As well as choosing local, raw honey you could opt for Manuka honey, which is harvested in New Zealand. It is renowned for its anti-bacterial strength which is graded according to its UMF, or unique Manuka factor. This denotes how high its anti-bacterial content is, so the higher the number the better. You want to aim for at least 10 on this scale.

Whether it's raw or Manuka, adding roughly a teaspoon a day to your diet is a good amount. Do avoid heating honey, however, as this reduces its health-giving properties. A couple of words of caution here, though: if you suffer from a history of anaphylactic reactions or have known sensitivities to bee pollen, royal jelly or any bee products then you need to pass. And for all those who are free to enjoy it, heed the words of Pooh Bear: 'I wasn't going to eat it, I was just going to *taste* it.' Too much of a good thing is never a good idea, so stick to just the one spoonful!

simply book a long holiday in the sunshine, as vitamin D is produced by daily exposure to the sun, though we're talking small daily doses here. It'll also give you a decent period of rest and relaxation – and the gut loves that too.

leaky gut

We have mentioned intestinal permeability or leaky gut a couple of times already so let's look at what it really means, the factors that can contribute to it and how to help restore and replenish a gut lining that has become permeable.

Intestinal permeability is a hot topic – and a controversial one – in nutrition and while the majority of research is currently linking this more specifically to gastrointestinal or immune conditions, there are also studies to suggest that it may have a role to play in gut health more generally, so I feel it is important to understand a bit more about it. Leaky gut doesn't sound pretty and it isn't. Think of the gut lining as a fine mesh that allows very small molecules and nutrients to pass seamlessly through. Now think of that same mesh with gaping holes in it. Not so good. The scientific term for this is intestinal permeability. The theory is that inflammation and irritation compromise the permeability of the lining, causing microscopic holes or tears that allow bacteria, foodstuffs and other foreign substances to pass through into the bloodstream. As I pointed out earlier, these 'alien invaders' should be kept within the safe confines of the gut wall so their escape triggers the immune system to mount an inflammatory response, and an often overzealous one, that can result in our own tissues getting caught in the crossfire. This is thought to be the link between leaky gut and autoimmune diseases, which we examined earlier in the chapter. However, leaky gut isn't solely related to autoimmune diseases. In fact, it has been associated with myriad conditions that include mood and anxiety disorders, irritable bowel disease, thyroid imbalances, food sensitivities and atopic allergies such as eczema, asthma and hay fever.

allergies and leaky gut

You may be surprised to hear that atopic allergies such as eczema (atopic dermatitis), hay fever (allergic rhinitis) and asthma can be caused by an overloaded immune system and a more permeable intestinal barrier. I often see clients who, in a desperate bid to resolve their symptoms, have visited countless specialists in these conditions, slapped on all sorts of creams and tried different medications or procedures, all to little or no lasting effect. Might they be missing the crucial underpinning factor in the functioning of the immune system? You guessed it, the gut!

These atopic allergies are by nature triggered by a disruption in the immune system. This means the immune system produces antibodies known as IgE (Immunoglobulin E) in response to an allergy, and it is these antibodies that stimulate certain cells to release inflammatory chemicals such as histamine. This then creates the associated response which, depending on the type of allergy, may, for instance, restrict breathing in asthma or create skin symptoms in the case of eczema. Studies show that patients with these allergic disorders have a lack of diversity in their microbiome and are also more likely to have had limited exposure to plenty of beneficial bacteria in infancy. This means fewer of these beneficial bacteria are able to thrive in the gut, which leads to a compromised microbiome and immune system and, potentially, a more permeable intestinal barrier.

Certain infections in the gut, for example *Candida albicans* (a type of yeast fungus), can also be prevalent in people who suffer from these allergic disorders because the fungus not only exacerbates the allergic response and disrupts the balance of microorganisms but, even more crucially, has a direct role in creating a more permeable lining by adhering to the intestinal barrier itself. That's why leaky gut may have some correlations with these types of allergies.

You can use the general suggestions on how to help restore a leaky gut on page 99, but if you have allergies you may also wish to run a food allergy test to see if these might be contributing to your condition. Note this is different from food intolerance. (We will look at the difference between the two in more detail in Chapter 6.)

the causes of leaky gut

anti-nutrients

Food, unsurprisingly, could be considered one of the key contributing factors in leaky gut. First, let's look at the influence of wheat and gluten. Gliadin and glutenins are the two main families of gluten proteins, which are found in wheat and other cereal grains. Essentially they give the grain that binding, sticky 'glue' factor. Coeliac disease, the condition that leads to severe malabsorption of nutrients, is a direct allergic response to these proteins. However, gliadin also activates zonulin, a protein that can allow the gut to become more permeable. This is actually a normal response and not too much of a problem if there are enough beneficial bacteria to maintain the gut wall, but when these bacteria are depleted or outnumbered by potential pathogens this initiates the release of more zonulin, potentially making the gut lining even more permeable.

This situation can escalate and essentially means that foods containing gluten, when eaten in excess, can directly contribute to a leaky gut, particularly if the microbiome is unbalanced and more so if someone has a genetic predisposition to autoimmune disease. Typically you will find gluten in wheat and other cereal grains, including most flours, bread, pasta and crackers, but it is also present in some less obvious sources, such as ketchup and mayo.

Gluten aside, the reality is that all grains, whether gluten-free or not, naturally contain 'anti-nutrient' compounds that are created by plants as a means of defence (well, they don't have teeth or claws). The intended effect is to make the animal (or human) ingesting them sick and less likely to come back for more. These toxic compounds can impair absorption of nutrients and create irritation and damage to the gut barrier. They include other proteins called lectins, organic acids known as phytates, saponins that have detergent-like properties, and enzyme inhibitors that impair our ability to break down food.

Grains are not the only food group to contain these anti-nutrients. Beans, pulses and legumes, such as lentils and chickpeas, as well as nuts and seeds, contain similar substances. The solution? Try to get into the habit of sprouting, soaking thoroughly and/or fermenting, which reduces most of these effects. Soaking beans from dried before cooking, for example, will make all their nutritional and gut-supportive nutrients more available, and they are super-nutritious foods after all! (Check out my useful soaking and sprouting chart on page 16.)

You can also opt for breads such as sourdough, which, although it still contains some gluten, is made from a fermentation process that negates many of the anti-nutrient properties. It therefore tends to be more digestive friendly for most people. You can also consider how grains, gluten-containing or not, have been cultivated. Pesticides and other sprays that we take in

When the gut is under constant stress and the defences have broken down, as in the case of leaky gut, you need to avoid taxing it further by feeding it stuff it could very happily do without.

through these foods could be a contributing factor in leaky gut (we will look at this topic in Chapter 10).

white, fried and dyed

Eating refined, sugary and highly processed foods in excess doesn't support the health of the microbiome and in turn can be one of the factors in leaky gut. A high intake of white, fried and dyed foods can give rise to certain microbes, such as yeasts and these can have a direct impact on the lining of the gut. Moreover they don't provide many of the nutrients, such as fibre, that our beneficial microorganisms need to thrive.

Now, reading this, you might be starting to tear your hair out but before you get hysterical about never having a piece of bread or a slice of cake again it's important to realise that this is all about the cumulative load of these trigger factors. The fact is that a lot of us unwittingly, or wittingly, expose ourselves to gluten and refined foods at every single meal. This overloads the gut and chronic inflammation can ensue. So the problem is not necessarily down to a particular food group per se but simply eating too much of these types of foods. A robust gut should be able to tolerate infrequent exposure to these foods and repair itself. However, when the gut is under constant stress and the defences have broken down, as in the case of leaky gut, you need to avoid taxing it further by feeding it stuff it could very happily do without.

other factors

As well as food, other factors can impair the lining of the gut, including excess alcohol, infections and medications such as antibiotics and anti-inflammatories. Furthermore, environmental toxins such as pesticides, food additives and preservatives, and even household cleaning products, all contribute to a general toxic overload that can have repercussions for the gut and the intestinal barrier. You can read more on these gut saboteurs in Chapters 7 and 10. Chronic stress is also a big factor so we'll look at the impact of a high-octane lifestyle on the gut in Chapter 8.

Infections such as *H. pylori* (the main cause of stomach ulcers) and small intestinal bacterial overgrowth (SIBO) may also contribute to a leaky gut due to the overgrowth of pathogens and too few beneficial bacteria to man the lining of the gut. (You'll find more info on this in Chapter 3.)

how to restore a leaky gut

If you think a leaky gut may be relevant to your gut health, I would encourage you to seek the support of a nutritional therapist so they can determine the best protocol for you. Nevertheless, you might wish to kick-off the process by stopping the cycle because leaky gut can be self-perpetuating. Once you start on an inflammatory loop it will simply keep going round and round until you press stop. You can begin by removing potential trigger foods such as gluten, wheat and grains (unless they have been soaked, sprouted or fermented to reduce the anti-nutrient substances they contain, and even then keep to a minimum amount initially). And, if you want to determine any additional factors that may be exacerbating the situation, work with your nutritional therapist, who can arrange a stool analysis to pinpoint potential bacterial imbalances and digestive deficiencies.

the magic of mushrooms

Love them or loathe them, when it comes to immune-boosting foods mushrooms are a headline act. 'Shrooms in all of their magical varieties have been used for hundreds of years for their medicinal properties. They are packed full of nutrition, providing B vitamins that help to support energy processes as well as many trace minerals such as selenium and copper. Depending on where they are grown they can provide a type of vitamin D, which is crucial for the immune system. They also contain a powerful antioxidant called ergothioneine that helps protect cells from damage.

However, it is in the compounds present in the cellular walls of mushrooms that things get really interesting. These consist of long sugar molecule chains known as polysaccharides and, within these, other active substances such as beta-glucans, proteins and enzymes. Extensive research has shown that these compounds have a significant impact on the immune system. The polysaccharides, for example, help to coordinate our immune cell 'troops', priming them to kill defunct cells. They also balance the two arms of T helper cells (see page 92), to give an even level of Th1 and Th2. This essentially means a more balanced immune system. Mushrooms also have an anti-bacterial and prebiotic effect on the microbiota in the gut by feeding beneficial bacteria while decreasing potential pathogens. There is a misconception that because they are fungi they automatically feed fungus in the gut, when in most cases they *compete* with other fungi and therefore have an anti-fungal effect.

So how do you get the best out of them? Technically any mushroom, even the simple button variety, has tons of nutritional value. But to really tap into the properties mentioned above, you need to go for the funkier types such as reishi, cordyceps, shiitake, oyster and enoki. Choose organic wherever possible, as mushrooms readily absorb chemicals from the soil. Dried is also a great option, particularly for some of the rarer varieties.

I've merely scratched the surface of the wondrous health benefits of mushrooms here, and I would highly recommend reading more – see page 271 for details of one of my favourite books on the subject.

what to eat

Eating plenty of gut-nourishing foods is just as, if not more, important as eliminating foods that can compromise the gut lining. Number one on the list should be bone broth, due to its collagen content and brilliant amino acid profile (particularly l-glutamine, a critical amino acid for the gut lining). Simmering the bones and ligaments to make the broth releases these healing compounds, which can help to restore the lining of the gut. So get those bones boiling, make up a big batch of broth and whack some into the freezer. I've provided a recipe for Chicken Bone Broth on page 57 and also used it as a base in a number of recipes, including my Carrot and Coconut Chermoula Soup (page 203) and Spicy Parsnip Satay Soup (page 83).

Fermented foods are also supportive as they provide natural sources of beneficial bacteria to help bolster the immune system. Try making my Mushroom, Miso and Manchego on Sourdough (page 102). It's quick, delicious and packs in three fermented heroes in the form of miso, Manchego and sourdough. Good quality fats found in food sources such as coconut oil, ghee, organic free range eggs, wild oily fish and avocados provide essential oils that help to reduce inflammation. My Nasi Goreng (page 107) and Wild Salmon with Butternut Rosemary Purée and Crispy Kale (page 134) are super-tasty dishes brimming with healthy oils. Raw honey can also help, due to the immune-supportive properties that were mentioned earlier.

There are also certain supplements that can help this process, including a good probiotic, digestive enzymes and an l-glutamine powder. We need large amounts of l-glutamine, particularly to help restore the gut lining, and although it is always better to get this from your food as much as possible, it may be helpful to supplement.

Finally, it's not just about targeting physical 'stressors'. A huge part of supporting a healthy gut barrier comes from reducing or eliminating external stress as well. You need to prioritise those precious moments of recovery – whether that's taking up a gentle yoga practice, doing a Pilates class, meditating or simply setting aside time to read. Such moments of rest are vital in assisting the gut to repair and regenerate.

value your defences

You can now appreciate why the health of the immune system is so inherently dependent on the gut, and how through supporting a healthy gut we maintain a robust natural armour. Our internal army depends on giving the gut the ammunition and reserves it needs to function at its best, and that relies on feeding it the right foods and nutrients. The recipes that follow complement the information in this chapter but that doesn't mean they fall short on taste. So while you are boosting your reserves you can also eat with a real sense of satisfaction.

blueberry and sprouted buckwheat bircher muesli

When it comes to eating grains, it is a question of which types of grains can best support gut health. Sprouting removes some of the 'anti-nutrient' substances – the grains' natural defensive shield, which can impair absorption – and allows us to access all their bountiful health benefits. Sprouted buckwheat has a lovely crunchy texture and soaking it overnight brings out even more of its flavour and nutritional virtues. Chia seeds are a great plant-based source of omega 3 – important for its anti-inflammatory properties – and they give this recipe a richer consistency. The addition of vanilla and punchy blueberries provides a naturally sweet start to the day.

serves 1

80g sprouted buckwheat

2 tablespoons chia seeds

200ml milk (choose from: full fat organic unhomogenised dairy milk, raw if you can get it, unsweetened cashew or almond milk or full fat coconut milk)

Seeds from ½ vanilla pod or ¼ teaspoon vanilla powder

Dash fresh lemon juice

Generous handful blueberries

Mix all of the ingredients, except the blueberries, together in a small bowl or glass tumbler and place in the fridge overnight.

In the morning, remove from the fridge 5–10 minutes before you want to eat, adding a little additional milk if needed. Top with blueberries.

tip
Swap the buckwheat for sprouted oats if you prefer.

mushroom, miso and manchego on sourdough

The three Ms here make a pretty mean combo. Miso and Manchego are both excellent natural sources of beneficial bacteria and mushrooms help those bacteria to find a happy home in the gut. This fierce trio sitting on top of the king of fermented bread that is sourdough makes this a brilliant option for when you need a tasty lunch that is filling, bursting full of gut-friendly foods and best of all takes next to no time to make. Cheese on toast just got pimped up!

serves 1

2 slices fresh sourdough

1 tablespoon unpasteurised miso paste

¼ teaspoon mild mustard powder

2 tablespoons coconut aminos

6 shiitake or other mushrooms

1 teaspoon organic unsalted butter or ghee

7–8 fine shavings of unpasteurised Manchego

Pinch mineral-rich salt

Fresh oregano to serve

Preheat a grill to medium heat or use a toaster to lightly toast the sourdough.

Mix together the miso paste, mustard powder and 1 tablespoon of the coconut aminos in a small bowl.

Prepare the mushrooms by brushing them clean and then slicing. Heat the butter or ghee in a shallow pan and stir-fry the mushrooms for about 5 minutes, adding the remaining tablespoon of coconut aminos. Remove from the heat.

Place the toast on a plate and spread the miso mixture over the sourdough. Top with the mushrooms and then grate fine shavings of Manchego over the top. Finish with a pinch of salt and the fresh oregano.

cauli 'polenta' with shimeji and hazelnuts

Making polenta from cauliflower was a real discovery for me; roasted in the oven it gives a flavoursome take on traditional cornmeal polenta. Cauliflower, like other cruciferous veggies, such as cabbage and broccoli, contains compounds such as sulforaphane that are great for your gut and its many microbes. Mushrooms are excellent prebiotics that help to bolster your beneficial bacteria army and support a more robust immune system. This isn't just a nutritional feast for the gut: the deep cheesy taste, whether it's from Parmesan or yeast flakes, makes it a truly satisfying dish for our taste buds too. Plus it's a simple and quick supper option when you crave a really hearty and healthy meal at the end of a long day.

serves 2

1 cauliflower, cut into small florets

4 garlic cloves, peeled and crushed

1 small onion, peeled and quartered

4 tablespoons extra virgin olive oil, plus a little extra to finish

4 tablespoons grated Parmesan or other unpasteurised hard cheese (or substitute 6 tablespoons (20g) nutritional yeast flakes for a vegan version)

Mineral-rich salt and black pepper

Juice of ½ lemon

8–10 button mushrooms

150g shimeji mushrooms (or use other mushrooms, such as shiitake)

1 tablespoon organic unsalted butter or ghee (use coconut oil for a vegan version)

4–6 tablespoons coconut aminos

Small cupped handful hazelnuts, lightly toasted, then lightly crushed

Fresh herbs, finely chopped (chervil or flat-leaf parsley works best)

Preheat the oven to 200°C/Gas 6. Line a baking tray or ovenproof dish with baking parchment. Place the cauliflower, garlic and onion on the lined tray and roast for about 25 minutes until tender. (If you haven't already toasted the hazelnuts, you can add them for the last 5 minutes of cooking.)

Add the roasted cauliflower, onion and garlic to a food processor. Then add the olive oil, Parmesan (or yeast flakes), a few decent pinches of salt and pepper and the lemon juice and a touch of filtered water to thin as desired. Pulse until you have a smooth, creamy, polenta-like texture.

To cook the mushrooms, heat the butter, ghee or coconut oil in a frying pan, add all the mushrooms and cook on a medium heat for about 5 minutes. Add the coconut aminos and cook for a further minute. Remove from the heat.

To serve, divide the cauliflower mix between two plates, spoon the mushroom mix on top, then add the hazelnuts, drizzle with a touch more olive oil and garnish with fresh herbs.

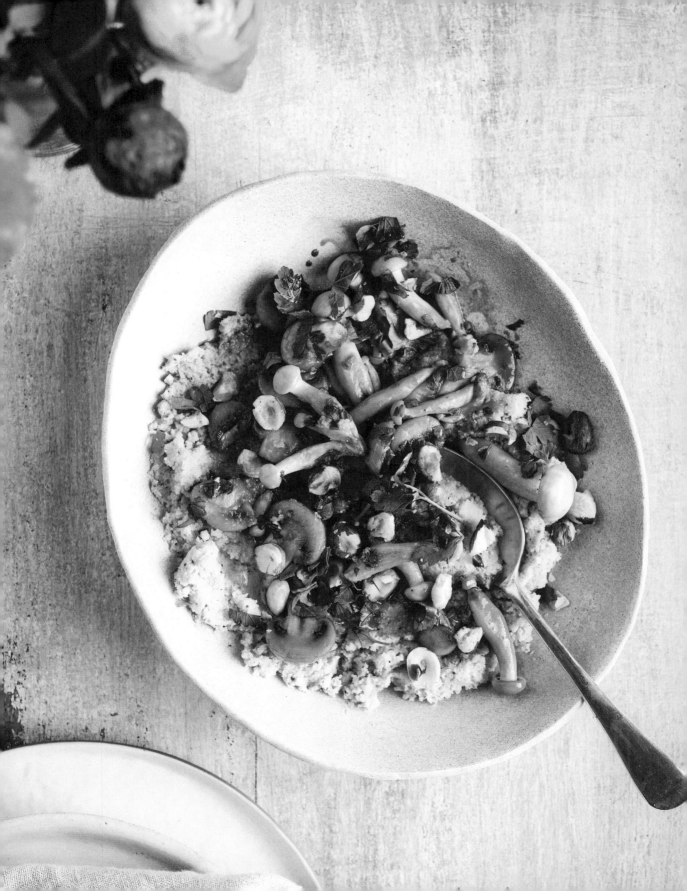

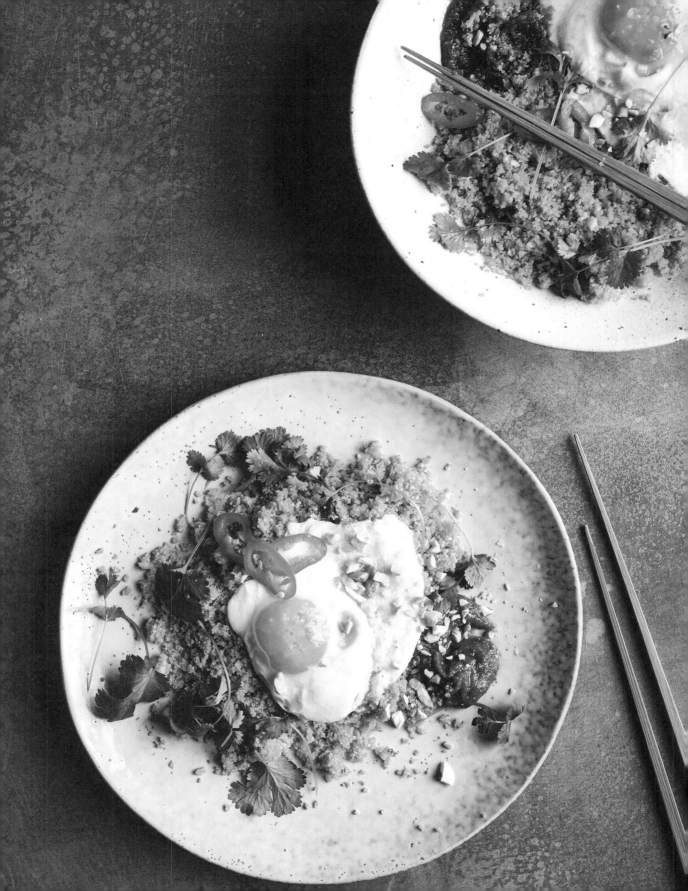

nasi goreng

Once you start making cauliflower 'rice' you will soon realise just how incredibly easy and quick it is and, even more importantly, how great it tastes. It is a member of the cruciferous vegetable family, so it also packs a serious nutritional punch, providing lots of natural gut and detoxification support. Paired with the vibrant spices of this classic Indonesian dish and finished with a cheery fried egg, it will make you and your gut smile.

serves 2

1 teaspoon coconut oil

2 organic free range eggs (or substitute 150g non-GMO tempeh for a vegan version)

1 teaspoon organic unsalted butter or ghee (or coconut oil for a vegan version)

Handful fresh coriander leaves

6 fine slices fresh chilli

1 tablespoon crushed cashews (optional)

cauliflower 'rice'

1 cauliflower

Pinch chilli powder

½ teaspoon garlic powder

1 teaspoon onion powder

2 teaspoons ground galangal

2 teaspoons ground cumin

2 teaspoons ground turmeric

¼ teaspoon ground cardamom

6 dried lime leaves

3 tablespoons desiccated coconut

2 generous pinches mineral-rich salt

Generous pinch black pepper

sambal sauce

3 tablespoons tomato paste

Pinch chilli powder

2 teaspoons mild smoked paprika

2 teaspoons onion powder

Generous pinch mineral-rich salt

To prepare the cauliflower rice, place all the ingredients in a food processor and pulse until you have a rice-like texture.

Mix all of the sambal sauce ingredients together and add a tablespoon of filtered water to thin. Place in the fridge.

Heat the coconut oil in a saucepan on a low heat and cook the cauliflower rice for 2–3 minutes.

Meanwhile, fry your eggs (or tempeh) in butter, ghee or coconut oil. I like to keep the yolk runny so it oozes into the rice, but cook to your liking.

When the rice is cooked, divide between two plates, top with the eggs and add a generous tablespoon of the sambal sauce. Garnish with the coriander leaves, chilli slices and crushed cashews if desired.

sweet potato and warm halloumi salad with tahini dressing

Sweet potatoes provide a wealth of nutritional benefits: they are high in beta-carotene, which is important for our skin and immune health, and are a great source of fibre for our gut microbes. Halloumi, like other ewes' milk cheeses, tends to be easier on digestion for most. The combination of fresh mint and dill adds a vibrant colour, and fresh herbs are brilliant for flavour and for the gut.

serves 2

1 large sweet potato, peeled and cut into chunks

1 tablespoon organic unsalted butter or ghee

4 slices (90g) unpasteurised halloumi, cut into 12–15 cubes

Small handful fresh mint leaves, roughly chopped

2 tablespoons chopped fresh dill

3 tablespoons tahini

Juice of 1 lemon

2 generous pinches mineral-rich salt

4 tablespoons extra virgin olive oil

Preheat the oven to 200°C/Gas 6. Line a baking tray with baking parchment. Put the sweet potato on the baking tray and cook for 25–30 minutes until tender.

While the sweet potato is cooking, heat a small frying pan on a medium heat, add the butter or ghee and lightly fry the halloumi for 4–6 minutes, stirring occasionally, until golden. Remove from the heat and place in a bowl.

Add the mint and dill to the bowl with the halloumi.

For the dressing, mix the tahini, lemon juice, salt, 2 tablespoons of the olive oil and a little filtered water to thin; put to one side.

When the sweet potato is cooked, remove from the oven and add to the bowl with the halloumi, mint and dill and combine all together. Transfer to a serving plate and drizzle with the dressing and the remaining 2 tablespoons of olive oil.

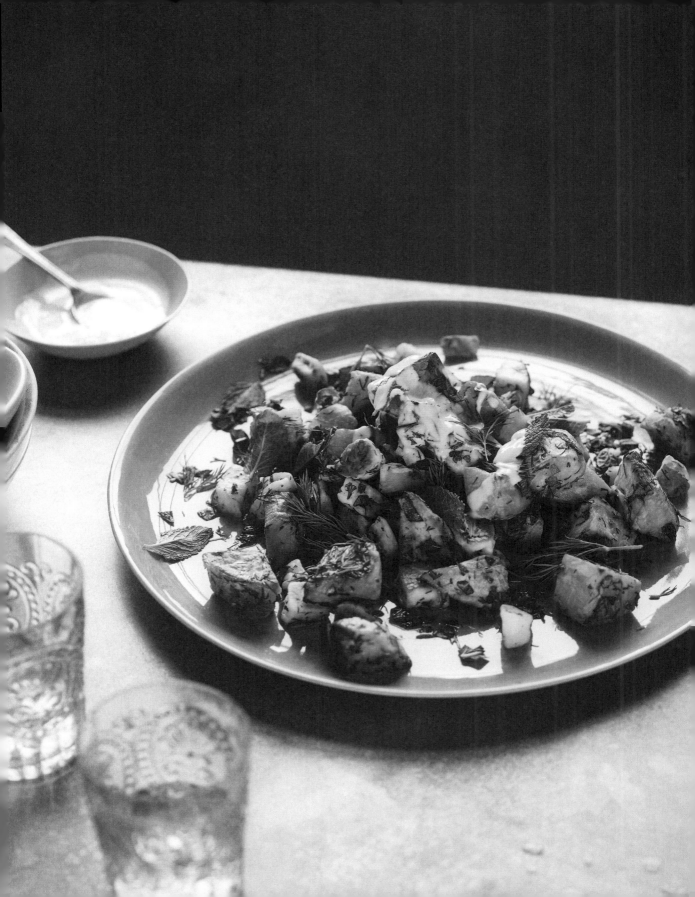

sea bass with turmeric corn polenta

As a kid I loved a buttery corn on the cob and sweetcorn works brilliantly as a polenta, with a sweeter taste than the more usual dried cornmeal; it is also less irritating to the gut and overall much more nutritious. With a touch of turmeric that gives a deep golden colour and also helps to support our gut immune army, it goes beautifully with white fish, along with fragrant marjoram. I have specified line-caught sea bass, and would always try to source fish that has been caught sustainably, as stocks are severely depleted. You can substitute another white fish, but make sure it is on the list of sustainable fish published by the Marine Stewardship Council (MSC) and always look for the blue MSC label.

serves 2

2 fillets line-caught sea bass, descaled, approx. 90g per fillet

200g frozen sweetcorn

2 tablespoons fresh lemon juice

2 tablespoons extra virgin olive oil, plus extra to drizzle

1 teaspoon ground turmeric

¼ teaspoon garlic powder

Generous pinch mineral-rich salt and black pepper

1 tablespoon organic unsalted butter or ghee

Leaves from 3 sprigs marjoram or oregano

Run your fingers lightly over the sea bass fillets to make sure there are no bones.

Cook the sweetcorn, ideally in a steamer. Drain and then add to a high-speed blender with the lemon juice, olive oil, turmeric, garlic powder, salt and pepper. Blend until smooth.

In a frying pan, heat the butter or ghee on a high heat. Season the fish with a little salt and pepper just before cooking. Add the fillets skin side down and press them down with a spatula (or carefully with your fingers) to stop them curling. Reduce the heat to medium and leave the fish to cook – without touching or moving it – for 3–4 minutes until the flesh is almost cooked and the skin starts to crisp. Flip over and cook on the flesh side for 2 minutes.

While the fish is cooking, divide the polenta between two plates. Top with the sea bass, drizzle with a little olive oil and scatter over some fresh marjoram or oregano.

stewed cinnamon apples with raw honey kefir cream

The saying 'an apple a day' certainly has its merits, specifically when it comes to the gut. Apples contain a type of fibre called pectin, which helps to feed the beneficial microbes in the gut so they can produce anti-inflammatory substances; when stewed, apples more easily release their pectin. Here they are served with a raw honey kefir cream that provides additional probiotic benefits and an immune boost. Ideally make the cream at least an hour in advance so that it has time to set. I love this as a sumptuous gut-supportive breakfast. A smaller serving of the raw honey kefir cream is also delicious with my Hazelnut, Cardamom and Cacao Granola (page 174).

serves 2

2 red or green dessert apples

2 teaspoons ground cinnamon

¼ teaspoon ground cardamom

1 teaspoon fresh thyme leaves

2 heaped tablespoons flaked almonds

raw honey kefir cream

160g cashews, soaked for 2 hours, drained and rinsed

100ml kefir (dairy or coconut)

1 tablespoon tahini

1 tablespoon raw honey

1 teaspoon vanilla extract

Pinch mineral-rich salt

First make the kefir cream: put all the ingredients into a high-speed blender and blend on high until you have a smooth cream. You will need to use the tamper to push down the ingredients, or stop and scrape a few times. Transfer to a sealable glass or ceramic container, place in the fridge and leave to set. It is best if you make this a few hours in advance.

Core the apples, then cut into quarters and cut in half again, so you have eight pieces from each apple. Put the apples in a saucepan with 3 tablespoons of filtered water, the cinnamon, cardamom and thyme. Bring to the boil, lower the heat to a simmer and cover the pan. Simmer for about 5 minutes until the apples soften and the skin becomes shiny.

Divide the apples between two plates and add the flaked almonds. Serve with a scoop of the kefir cream for each plate.

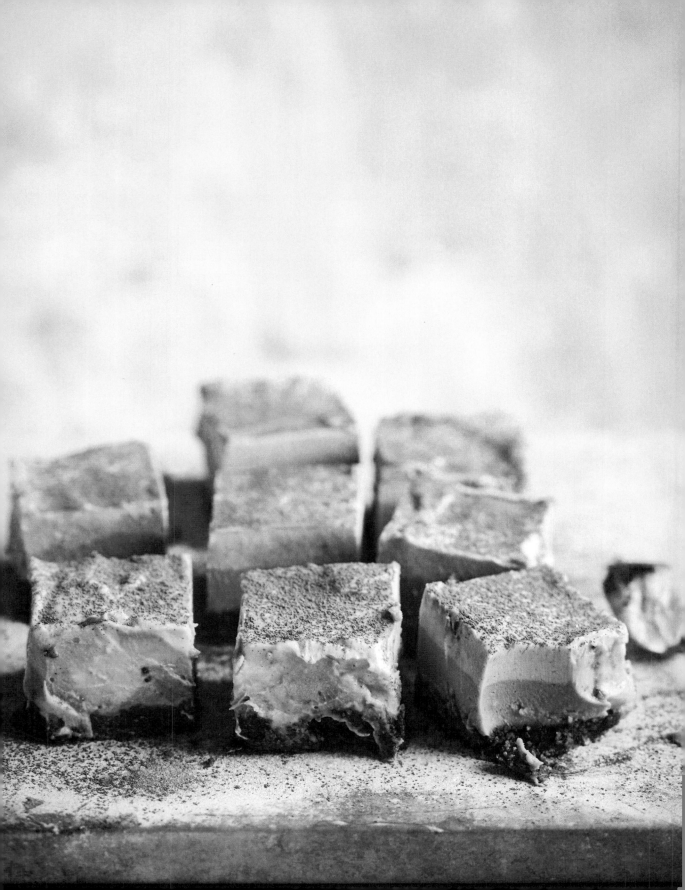

tirami-shroom

Tiramisu is one of my all-time favourite desserts, so I had a lot of fun creating this more gut-friendly version. Mushroom extract might seem an odd ingredient, but it lifts the coffee flavour to another level and gives your gut army a boost too. My shopping guide (page 263) has info on where you can buy this. I have used coconut blossom nectar as a sweetener because raw honey (my usual choice of sweetener) tastes a bit strong in this recipe. Coconut blossom has few of the negative health issues associated with some of the other, supposedly 'healthy', sugar substitutes, such as agave nectar – and after all this is meant to be a treat. It's perfect with a hot steaming cup of joe.

You will need to 'activate' your almonds and sunflower seeds by soaking and drying them (see page 16) and this must be done at least 24 hours in advance, but you can make bigger batches and store them ready to use in other recipes or to eat as a snack.

makes 1 cake (approx. 16 servings)

vanilla cream

200ml full fat coconut milk

190g cashews, soaked for 2 hours, drained and rinsed

20g desiccated coconut

Seeds from 2 vanilla pods

Pinch mineral-rich salt

coffee cream

1 shot espresso or 4 tablespoons strong filtered coffee

200ml full fat coconut milk

315g cashews, soaked for 2 hours, drained and rinsed

2 teaspoons mushroom extract

Pinch mineral-rich salt

almond base

150g activated almonds with skins

30g activated sunflower seeds

25g cacao nibs

Seeds from 1 vanilla pod

1 tablespoon mushroom extract

¼ teaspoon mineral-rich salt

1 shot espresso or 4 tablespoons strong filtered coffee

3 tablespoons coconut blossom nectar

A little raw cacao powder to serve

method overleaf

tirami-shroom method

To make the vanilla cream, put all the ingredients into a high-speed blender and blend until smooth and creamy; use a tamper to push down the ingredients, or stop and scrape a few times. Transfer to a ceramic or glass bowl and place in the fridge. Rinse the blender thoroughly.

Make the coffee cream in the same way as the vanilla cream. Transfer to a separate ceramic or glass bowl and place in the fridge.

To make the almond base, put the almonds, sunflower seeds, cacao nibs, vanilla, mushroom extract and salt in a food processor and pulse until the mixture is like textured flour. Then add the coffee and coconut blossom nectar to bind.

Ideally, use a 15cm square baking tin with a removable base, which makes it easy to remove the cake from the tin. Otherwise, line a 15cm square tin with baking parchment so you can lift the cake

out when it comes to serving. First add the almond mixture, using the back of a metal spoon to press it evenly across the base of the tin. Next add the coffee cream in an even layer. Place in the freezer for around 30 minutes until set.

Top with an even layer of the vanilla cream and put back in the freezer for at least another 30 minutes. Remove from the freezer around 45 minutes before you wish to eat.

Just before serving, lightly dust with a little cacao powder, shaking it through a sieve.

tip

If you are not serving it straight away, you can keep it in the freezer for up to 1 month (you will need to cover it).

avocado 'nutella' cream

I created this as a healthier version of the original stuff, but once you get a taste of it you won't go back. Avocados are brimming full of healthy oils as well as B vitamins and fibre, which all help to support the functioning of the gut. What's more, it is sweetened with whole dates, which provide additional fibre for our gut microbes. Enjoy a scoop of this on it's own for dessert, use it to top porridge or spread it on toasted sourdough. For an extra decadent breakfast serve it alongside my Chocolate Chia Fudgy Pancakes with Coconut Vanilla Kefir (page 81).

6–8 servings

1 avocado
Seeds from 1 vanilla pod or 3–4 drops vanilla extract
35g cacao powder
5–6 pitted dates
3 tablespoons unsweetened hazelnut butter
2 tablespoons unsweetened coconut yogurt
Generous pinch mineral-rich salt
175–200ml filtered water

Place all the ingredients, with 150ml of the water, in a high-speed blender and blend on the highest setting, gradually adding a little more water until smooth and creamy (you may not need all the water).

Transfer to a sealable glass or ceramic container and store in the fridge for up to 3–4 days.

tip
Top with some activated hazelnuts to bring out even more of its nutty flavour.

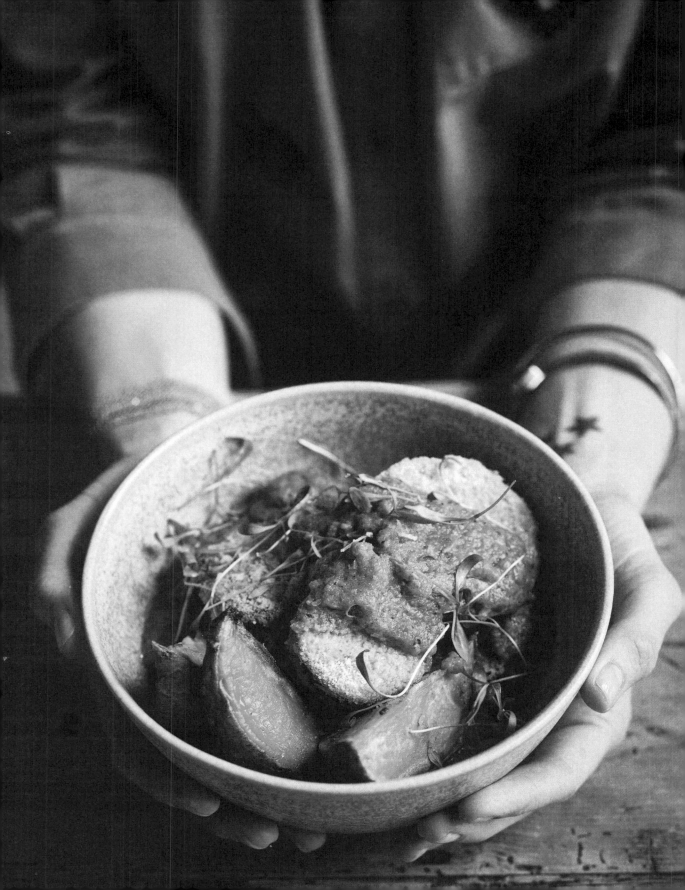

5

mind over matter

DO YOU EVER get the feeling of knowing something before you actually know it? Do you sometimes get an inexplicable compulsion to act on a certain feeling? Maybe you get a weird tingle, sweaty palms or queasiness in your stomach. Whatever it is that gives you that 'gut instinct' these are all real sensations that help us tune in to our innate wisdom.

The relationship between the gut and the brain epitomises the concept of a mind–body connection. We are certainly all familiar with the sensation of butterflies in the stomach: whether it's getting the jitters about a big work presentation or the anticipated excitement of meeting a loved one, it is a physical manifestation of emotions that you feel deep in your gut – a 'gut reaction'.

That core connection between the gut and brain is a real and mutually beneficial biochemical relationship that involves the nervous system and the many microbes that live in the gut.

This chapter reveals that a happy gut and a happy mind are fundamentally intertwined. Caring for your microbiome can have a huge impact on how you think and feel, so we'll look at the foods and factors that help to support this process. The recipes at the end of the chapter will help you put the information into practice through dishes such as my creamy Chicken, Almond and Celery Ballotine (page 137), quick and fun Green Eggs and Ham (page 132), and Popeye's Smoothie Bowl (page 127), which will add a boost of green veg to your brekkie. So get your thinking cap on: you might just learn to trust your 'gut instinct' a whole lot more after reading this.

the second brain

We have a highly complex organ in our head called the brain. Our grey matter is filled with billions of communicators called 'neurons' and it is these electrically excitable cells that transmit information to other cells in the body. On a day-to-day basis they manage thought processes such as focus and decision-making, as well as emotional wellbeing. However, the brain is not the only place in the body with 'thinking' potential. Yes, you guessed it, your gut also has its own intelligence system. I'll try to explain this as simply as I can.

Your gut 'brain' is called the enteric nervous system (ENS). It is part of the peripheral nervous system (PNS), which is basically the portion of the nervous system that is outside of the central nervous system (CNS) – your brain and spinal cord. Within the peripheral nervous system there are two divisions: the somatic nervous system (SNS), which deals with voluntary movements such as walking and smiling, and the autonomic nervous system (ANS), which regulates involuntary processes such as your heart beating, breathing and digestion. The enteric nervous system is therefore generally considered a subdivision of the autonomic nervous system – because we don't have to consciously think and send signals to make most of our digestive processes happen. Now that would be exhausting!

The enteric nervous system itself is made up of a highly complex array of nervous tissue that surrounds the entire gut and directly controls the gastrointestinal system. And while it does have considerable help from the rest of the autonomic nervous system, the enteric nervous system is able to function independently of the central nervous system, which is why it has been called 'the second brain'.

Within the enteric nervous system there are believed to be between 200 and 600 million neurons, more than in the spinal cord. These neurons in the gut largely communicate with the central nervous system through the vagus nerve, which meanders from the brain right down to the lowest part of the abdomen, interacting with other organs en route, such as the heart. This is the main channel of communication from the gut to the brain and vice versa, which means it constantly updates the brain on what is going on in the body. You might like to think of your 'gut feelings' as a stream of info from the gut to the brain via this channel. The brain also uses this feedback system to send signals that let the body know when it is time to 'rest and digest' or, if there is a perceived dangerous threat, activate the 'fight or flight' stress response. What's more, it isn't just neurons that influence this communication; microbes in the gut use the same vagus channel (we will come back to this shortly).

Just like the brain, the enteric nervous system relies on special chemical messengers called neurotransmitters that communicate between neurons and other cells in the body. There are many different neurotransmitters, including: serotonin, dubbed the 'happy hormone', the lack of which has been linked to depression and mood disorders, and which most anti-depressant medications target; dopamine, which is used for movement coordination and is related to feelings of motivation and

As most of our serotonin is made in the gut, an imbalance of bacteria may result in our gut failing to produce adequate amounts of serotonin. Essentially an unhappy gut leads to an unhappy mind.

pleasure; and GABA (gamma-amino butyric acid), a calming chemical that has an inhibitory effect on cell activity while glutamate has the opposite excitatory effect. There are also stress- and sleep-related neurotransmitters such as noradrenaline and adrenaline that are closely linked with the 'fight or flight' response.

The general assumption is that because these neurotransmitters are related to cognitive processes they are exclusively produced in the brain. Surprisingly, 90–95 per cent of our serotonin is manufactured in the gut, as is a large proportion of some of these other chemicals. So let's investigate how this happens and why the microbes in the gut have such a significant role to play in how we think and feel.

it's all in your head … or is it?

In recent years mental health problems have skyrocketed. It is estimated that around one in four people in the UK will experience a mental health issue in any given year and with depression a major cause of disability worldwide it's no wonder that some of the most prescribed meds are anti-depressants. However, recent research has highlighted just how significant a role the gut has to play in all our cognitive processes. Given their direct physical links, it isn't really surprising that the

brain and the nervous system are so heavily influenced by the health of the gut. This means that to resolve an issue we may have thought was all in our head, we might need to adopt a much more holistic approach and take our gut health into account too.

In the previous section I introduced those clever messenger chemicals called neurotransmitters. Now I'll explain in more detail how the gut and more specifically the microbiome are so critically important in their production. In Chapter 4 we saw how important it is to maintain a healthy balance of bacteria in the gut for overall digestive health, but when that balance is off kilter it also interferes with the production of neurotransmitters, including serotonin. As most of our serotonin is made in the gut, a compromised microbiome may result in the gut failing to produce adequate amounts of serotonin. Essentially an unhappy gut leads to an unhappy mind.

What's worse is that this can lead to a seriously sad feedback loop, in that the more the microbiome is compromised, the fewer positive neurotransmitters are produced. This means that you are less able to deal with stress, which creates a cascade of inflammation, leading to further dysbiosis in the gut. And so the cycle goes around, again and again, further jeopardising our ability to manufacture these positive chemicals.

Changes in the integrity of the gut can also impair the working of the brain. That's why the health of the gut and the microbiota is so paramount. Gut–neurological dysfunction is often indicated in conditions such as Alzheimer's, Parkinson's, multiple sclerosis, depression and anxiety. One of the key markers of intestinal permeability or leaky gut are large particles called lipopolysaccharides (LPSs), which cannot cross the gut lining unless the intestinal barrier is compromised; these have been shown to be elevated in some neurological conditions. A leaky gut also allows pro-inflammatory chemicals, such as lipopolysaccharides and cytokines from the immune system, to circulate around the entire body – including the brain. This could explain why there is often a link between chronic inflammation, leaky gut and depression in conditions such as IBS and autoimmune diseases. It seems that leaky gut can lead to a leaky brain.

However, our gut does a lot more than simply manage the production of neurotransmitters. Compelling recent studies are pointing towards strains of bacteria that can produce chemicals that are identical to our own neurotransmitters. Some of the most prevalent anti-depressant medications, SSRIs (serotonin-specific reuptake inhibitors), are designed to alter neurotransmitter activity in the brain, not the gut, so this fascinating research could in the future have a place in helping to manage certain types of depression and anxiety.

Our trillions of microbes also have a role to play in producing brain-derived neurotrophic factor (BDNF), a protein that is crucial for the health of the neurons in the brain. Gut bacteria supply most of our vitamin B_{12}, which is critical for our neurological health: deficiency is often associated with increased risk of dementia and depression. And certain strains in the *Bifidobacterium* family seem to make tryptophan (the precursor to serotonin) more available for the body to absorb. Indeed, those suffering with depression tend to show lower levels of tryptophan.

In addition, bacteria, like neurons, use the vagus nerve to communicate with the brain. In this way, they may influence what we choose to eat by driving certain cravings. From an evolutionary point of view this would be a smart move, as it would allow their species to flourish in the gut. These gut bugs are much more intelligent than we think!

It is mind-blowing to think that you can actually change the way you feel by changing the environment for the bacteria in your gut. By cultivating a more diverse microbiome you have the potential to have a more 'friendly' output of feel-good substances and manage inflammation better. By nourishing the bacteria in your gut, you are nourishing your mind.

feed your mind

So now that we understand just how important the gut is to the functioning of the brain, let's look at how to support a healthy mind through feeding the gut and all its healthy microbes the foods they'll love.

carbs

Let's talk carbohydrates, or carbs, first. In recent years there has been a lot of confusion about carbs: they have either been vilified (by advocates of certain types of high-protein

turmeric

When it comes to antioxidants and their protective roles, turmeric is a winner. This beautiful golden spice has been revered in India for centuries for its health-promoting properties but it is only fairly recently that scientific research has revealed why turmeric is so beneficial. Its power is derived from naturally occurring chemical compounds, the most significant being curcumin, which gives it all of its incredible molecular benefits. Curcumin has a justifiable reputation as a potent anti-inflammatory: research shows that it targets and blocks a molecule that switches on inflammatory mediators and has been linked to chronic diseases and neurological conditions.

As a potent antioxidant, this punchy powerhouse helps to protect the body from damaging free radicals (molecules that can damage cells); along with neutralising these substances it boosts our own production of natural antioxidant enzymes. Curcumin may also have neurocognitive benefits due to its positive influence on BDNF, a chemical produced within the body that is linked to the protection of neurons. It also helps support the metabolism of amyloid plaque, which can best be described as a sticky build-up of proteins in the brain that has been linked to Alzheimer's and dementia. Finally, turmeric also assists with managing our immune system, where its intracellular actions seem to support a healthy turnover of cells and apoptosis (natural cell death).

For the body to get the optimum benefit from it, turmeric needs a partner in crime in the form of black pepper; this supports its absorption and is probably why the two taste so good together. And because it's fat-soluble, turmeric is best eaten with some kind of healthy oil. This combo is a natural in curry. My Turmeric Chai Latte (page 211) is also a delicious way to give your brain and gut a boost. This superstar spice gets a gold medal every time.

diet) or eaten to excess, particularly the white, fried and dyed types. Our bodies, including our brains, need a certain amount of carbs to function properly – but not in the mass quantities and junk-food form that many of us gravitate towards. Yes, I'm talking about refined grains, high amounts of sugar and nutritionally devoid foods that give your blood sugar levels a rollercoaster ride and do nothing to support a healthy microbiome or a healthy mind either.

The brain naturally loves foods that are high in sugar and fat for the instant glucose gratification and the abundance of calories they provide.

After all, it is a hungry organ and needs a lot of sustenance: almost 20 per cent of our total carb intake goes to feed the brain. However, we can best support that natural inclination, and at the same time nourish the brain, by making a better choice with the types of carbohydrate we eat. The best way to do that is to choose the fibrous carbohydrates that our beneficial bacteria prefer. And that means vegetables in all their varieties (yes, in case you'd forgotten, vegetables contain carbs). Greens such as spinach, kale, chard, spring greens, cabbage, Brussels sprouts, broccoli and watercress not only provide fibre but also contain many of the important vitamins and minerals needed for neurotransmitter functioning. Other brain-boosting foods include cauliflower, beetroot, mushrooms, sprouted and/or fermented grains and sweet potatoes, as they also support our feel-good chemicals and contain protective antioxidants that prevent damage to cells.

And let's not forget the sources of resistant starches and prebiotics that provide our microbes with a feast: these include onions, raw garlic, leeks, asparagus, unripe bananas, Jerusalem artichokes and raw chicory root. As mentioned previously these prebiotics help our gut bacteria produce butyrate, a substance that is essential for the health of our colon cells. It also supports anti-inflammatory processes, which are linked to improved neurological health. In general the wider the variety of vegetables the better, as a diversity of nutrients and antioxidants cultivates a more diverse and plentiful microbiome. Fruits such as avocados, lemons, apples and berries are all excellent too.

protein

Our neurotransmitters entirely depend on amino acids to function, and amino acids are the building blocks of protein, so protein is critical for our brains to tick over nicely. For example, the amino acid tryptophan is the precursor of the neurotransmitter serotonin. And as we discovered at the start of the chapter, both of these amino acids are influenced and produced by microbes in the gut.

When it comes to protein, it is definitely a case of choosing quality over quantity. For example, organic grass-fed meats and free range poultry are not only more nutrient dense but have more of the anti-inflammatory omega 3 fats that the

In general the wider the variety of vegetables the better, as a diversity of nutrients and antioxidants cultivates a more diverse and plentiful microbiome.

brain needs. Oily fish such as salmon, sardines, pilchards, trout and mackerel are also rich in omega 3 (wild fish typically have higher levels than farmed fish). In general it's best to opt for smaller species of fish: larger fish such as swordfish and tuna have been found to contain heavy metals such as mercury, exposure to which has been linked to neurotoxicity. I'm not suggesting you avoid these fish completely, as they are an incredibly nutritious food source, but do think about the fish you buy and the amount you consume, as well as diversifying with other protein sources. Eggs are an excellent source of protein and choosing organic free range will give you more of a boost since they contain higher levels of omega 3 oils.

For vegan sources of protein, soaked and properly prepared legumes and pulses (see page 16 for my soaking chart) can be good choices. Nuts and seeds also contain plenty of protein, and they are also a rich source of fat, which leads us nicely on to the next part of feeding our brain …

fat

The brain is made up of 60 per cent fat. It's not the same type of fat as that stored in our bodies, but forms part of the make-up of the cell membranes and the myelin sheath that surrounds neurons. Because these neurons need to communicate effectively with each other, ensuring we get enough healthy fats into our diet is a big part of supporting brain health.

One of the richest sources of saturated fat found in nature is human breast milk, which is consumed at a time when a baby's brain is developing rapidly. It is the DHA (docosahexaenoic acid) component of breast milk that is the star of the show. DHA is an omega 3 fatty acid that makes up most of the brain and it has been found to be incredibly important in maintaining brain health throughout our lives. The best food sources are oily fish and algae (such as seaweed). The body can also convert the ALA (alpha-linolenic acid) omega 3 oils found in seeds and nuts into DHA; the best sources are flaxseed and chia seeds. Hemp seeds are another good way to increase your intake of ALA.

Walnuts – which even look rather like brains – are also great brain boosters. They contain the highest amount of omega 3 fats of any nut, again in the form of ALA, which has anti-inflammatory benefits. Walnuts also boast some 20 or more polyphenols, meaning they have high antioxidant properties.

The brain also needs other fats, such as the saturated fats found in unsalted organic butter, coconut oil and milk, as well as cold pressed oils such as extra virgin olive oil. Olive oil is a mainstay in the Mediterranean diet – a lifestyle associated with healthy longevity and a spritely mind – and is liberally drizzled over food at most meals. It also contains important polyphenol chemicals that support the brain and the gut.

probiotics

We looked at the benefits of natural probiotics in Chapter 2, and for the purpose of feeding the mind, foods that provide a direct source of beneficial bacteria also support a generally happier gut and brain.

Probiotic foods work in multiple ways to support better cognition. Firstly, they boost the beneficial bacteria that man the 'border checkpoint' of the gut in order to maintain the integrity of the intestinal barrier and prevent leaky gut. Remember, a leaky gut can lead to a leaky mind!

Probiotic foods also act like an enforcement agency, working with other bacteria in the gut to crowd out and actively evict those that create disruption and inflammation, another important aspect of supporting the brain. These bacteria also help us better absorb and indeed produce vitamins that we need to support neurotransmitter functioning.

Fermented foods are bursting with natural probiotics, and it is these types of foods that can give a boost to the gut. They include sauerkraut, kimchi, kefir, tempeh, miso, pickles, unpasteurised cheese and kombucha, a form of fermented tea that not only gives you a boost of probiotics but includes caffeine, which will stimulate your grey matter too (we'll come to that shortly). With all of these fermented beauties just make sure you choose those that are unpasteurised. With kefir, try to make your own from either raw milk (see page 153) or organic and unhomogenised full fat milk. You can also opt for a coconut version instead.

coffee and chocolate

Coffee and chocolate are good for you. Yes, you read that right. But before you get carried away, the type of coffee and chocolate, and the amount you drink and eat, are important. Anyone having 10+ espressos per day isn't going to be entirely sane, although some of my Italian friends may disagree. But when consumed in moderation, freshly ground coffee has been shown to have protective effects, particularly in relation to neurodegenerative conditions such as Alzheimer's and Parkinson's disease. Many of us recognise that surge of energy and brainpower after a cup of joe. However, some people are genetically predisposed not to tolerate caffeine well and for them a cup of coffee means a bad headache and an upset stomach, rather than a positive zing. But if you don't suffer from these unpleasant side effects then having a fresh cup each day can benefit your brain.

Chocolate doesn't give the same buzz as caffeine, unless you eat a lot of it – and that buzz is down to the sugar more than anything else. But beneath that sumptuous exterior lie some pretty potent compounds, such as theobromine, which studies show helps with mood-related symptoms such as anxiety and depression. It also contains the chemicals phenylethylamine and anandamide, both of which are associated with feelings of love and joy. Yes, chocolate really does stimulate positive emotions as well as our taste buds.

However, I'm specifically referring to chocolate bars with at least 70–80 per cent cocoa, and to raw cacao powder. In its powdered form cocoa is right at the top of the ORAC (Oxygen Radical Absorbance Capacity) scale, a measure of the level of antioxidants foods contain. It is worth investing in good quality chocolate with a high cocoa content. Cheaper choc won't have the same effect – the cocoa content is very low.

Both coffee and chocolate are also supportive for the gut due to their high flavonoid content. Flavonoids are powerful polyphenols, which means they have high antioxidant properties and as such play an important protective role throughout the body and not just in the gut. These same flavonoids also positively influence the gut microbiota, increasing the diversity of species and reducing less friendly organisms, such as clostridia, that can make you feel really unwell. So the good news is that a daily cup of fresh coffee and a square or two of good quality chocolate aren't simply giving you a boost; your gut microbes love them too.

shiny happy people

Having a positive frame of mind isn't solely about what you eat. Another key player in this picture is vitamin D. It's often referred to as the sunshine vitamin because the body creates this vital nutrient when we expose our skin to sunlight.

Vitamin D has a far-reaching influence on many processes in the body, including the nervous system and the brain. We know that there are vitamin D receptors in the brain and it has a significant role in supporting neurotransmitter and hormone functioning. Vitamin D also has a mutually beneficial relationship with our gut, so having adequate levels is critical for the health of the gut and brain.

The easiest way to get enough vitamin D is via exposure to the sun, but with modern lifestyles being very much indoors, deficiency is common. Even if you live in a hot climate you may not be getting enough because sunscreen creams limit the body's ability to synthesise vitamin D. Not that I'm advocating basking in the sun for hours on end, because the risk of skin cancer is serious, but it is important not to stay in the shade all the time. Experts reckon a daily exposure of 10 minutes outside of the hottest time of the day, without protection, is usually enough to keep your vitamin D levels topped up. If you think you may be deficient, you could try asking your GP for a blood test.

Vitamin D has a far-reaching influence on many processes in the body, including the nervous system and the brain.

you have brains in your head (and your gut!)

In the words of Dr Seuss, 'You have brains in your head. You have feet in your shoes. You can steer yourself any direction you choose.' In other words, each one of us is different. I have talked about the brain–gut connection, but by now you can see that it's really a microbiome–gut–brain connection. The microbes in the gut have a very active and indeed directional role in how we think, feel and behave. And they are steering us in many more ways than we might ever have imagined.

By feeding and enriching our beneficial bacteria with the right fuel we can enhance our mental capacity and performance. Feeding your brain with plenty of vegetables, good quality fats, oily fish and carefully chosen proteins can indeed help you to start thinking smarter and feeling better. Moreover, I defy anyone not to have a smile on their face after having a slice of my Matcha Banana Bread (page 128) or a taste of my Turmeric Chicken with Laksa Zoodles (page 135). Finding joy truly does begin with the food you are eating, particularly when it keeps your microbiome happy. Listen to your gut. It is telling you something.

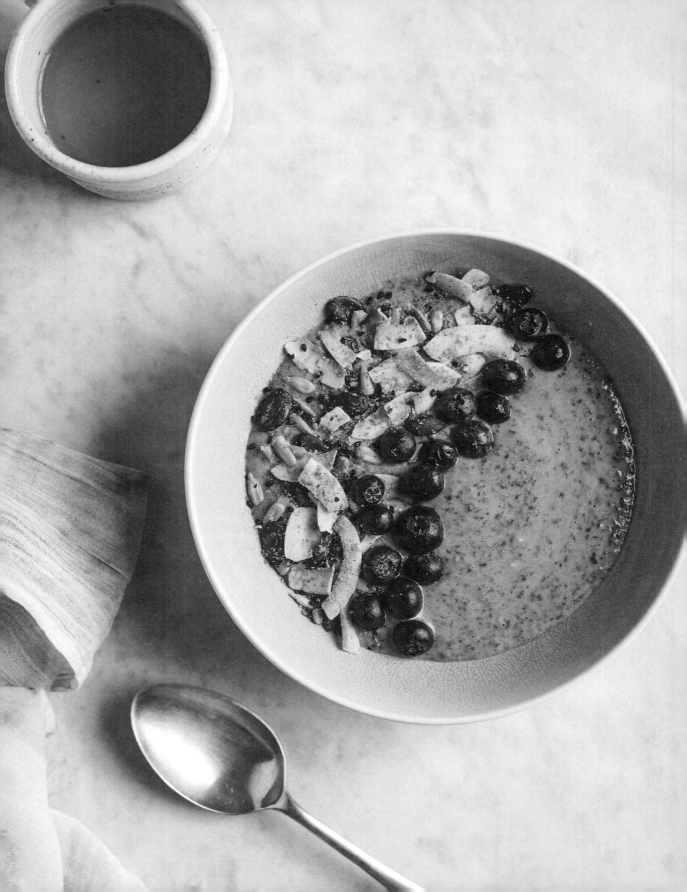

popeye's smoothie bowl with super seed mix

Having your smoothie in a bowl makes it more likely that you will sit down and eat it with a spoon rather than just knocking it back from a glass. And for optimum digestion we need to connect with the plate in front of us. This green machine of a recipe uses kale, spinach and avocado, which are packed with antioxidants to support the health of the gut and brain. The unripe banana provides resistant starch fibre, helping our gut microbes to produce crucial anti-inflammatory substances as well as serotonin, the 'happy hormone'. Maca powder helps the body to manage stress responses and it works well as a natural sweetener. You will need to 'activate' the seeds for the super seed mix (see page 16) and this must be done at least 24 hours in advance, but you can make bigger batches and store them to use in other recipes or as a snack.

serves 1

¼ avocado

1 unripe banana

1 handful spinach leaves

1 handful kale, stalks removed

1 pitted date

1 tablespoon unsweetened coconut yogurt

½ tablespoon almond nut butter

100ml unsweetened cashew or almond milk (or use raw or unhomogenised full fat organic dairy milk)

1 tablespoon maca powder

super seed mix

30g activated sunflower seeds

30g activated pumpkin seeds

3 tablespoons activated sesame seeds

3 tablespoons ground activated flaxseed

20g coconut chips

1 teaspoon coconut oil

Generous handful blueberries

Start by making the super seed mix. Preheat the oven to 150°C/Gas 2. Mix all of the seed ingredients in a bowl and spread over a baking tray. Bake for 15 minutes, then remove from the oven and leave to cool. Store in a sealable glass or ceramic container in the fridge for up to 3–4 weeks.

For the smoothie bowl, put all of the ingredients into a high-speed blender and blend to a creamy consistency.

Pour into a bowl and serve with 2 tablespoons of the super seed mix and a handful of blueberries.

tip

Buy frozen blueberries as they retain more nutritional value and you will have them conveniently to hand.

matcha banana bread

I'm a big fan of green tea and it doesn't get more potent than matcha. This green machine is a powdered version of green tea, from plants that are shaded from the sun for about three weeks before harvest. This increases the plant's natural chlorophyll levels, giving it a distinctive vibrant green colour. The veins and stems are removed, so you are ingesting only the leaves, making it a more potent form of green tea. And just like loose leaf green tea, the health benefits of matcha include high levels of polyphenols, antioxidants that have a protective effect and are great for our gut microbes. Matcha works particularly well in this banana bread that the whole family will enjoy tucking into; it's great for breakfast and it freezes well.

makes 1 loaf

1 tablespoon ground flaxseed
3 ripe bananas
3 tablespoons almond nut butter
Seeds from 2 vanilla pods
100ml unsweetened almond milk
50g coconut flour
25g ground almonds
25g flaked almonds
1 heaped tablespoon matcha
1 teaspoon bicarbonate of soda
1 tablespoon fresh lemon juice
Pinch mineral-rich salt

Preheat the oven to 180°C/Gas 4. Mix the flaxseed with 3 tablespoons of filtered water and set aside for 5 minutes.

In a large bowl, mash the bananas thoroughly and add the almond butter, soaked flaxseed, vanilla and almond milk and mix well.

Sift the coconut flour into a separate bowl and add the ground almonds, flaked almonds, matcha, bicarbonate of soda, lemon juice and salt and stir well. Add this mixture to the banana mix and combine well.

Line an 18 x 8cm loaf tin with baking parchment so that it hangs over the sides and scoop the mixture into the tin, spreading it evenly.

Bake for 1 hour. Lift up the baking parchment to remove the loaf and place it on a wire rack to cool. Slice and serve with either a spread of almond nut butter and raw honey or Raw Honey Kefir Cream (page 111).

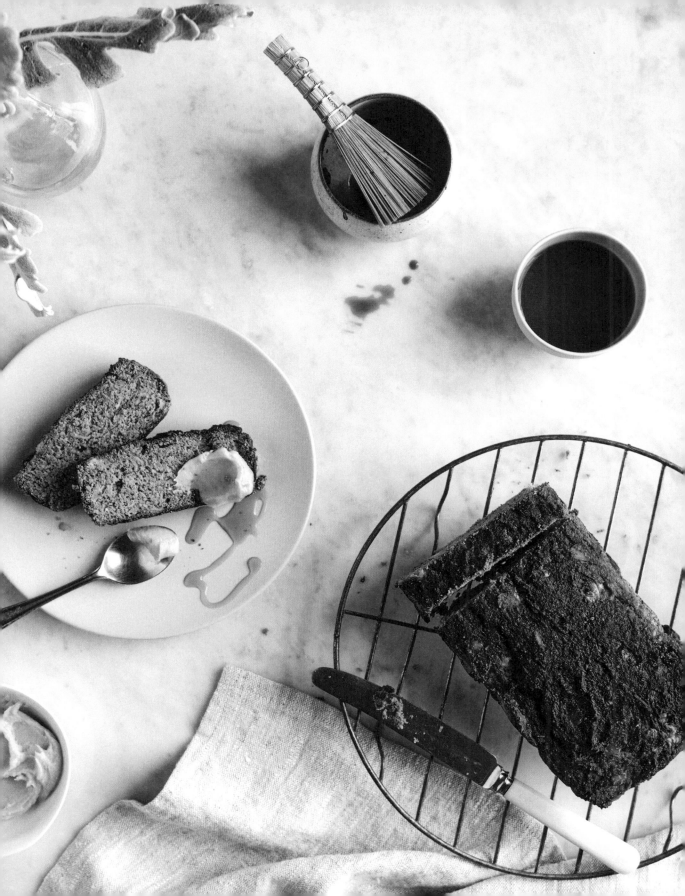

mackerel with beet and dill pickle salad

Mackerel is an oily fish with a high omega 3 content, important for its anti-inflammatory benefits and for supporting the health of our grey matter. The other ingredient that needs a shout out is beetroot. The bold colour of this purple veg comes from pigments known as betalains, antioxidants that help to negate any stressors in the body. They also support natural detoxification processes that give a helping hand to the gut. Their sumptuous flavour goes brilliantly with the richness of the mackerel in this easy and quick salad.

serves 2 (with extra beet salad)

2 medium beetroots (about the size of a tennis ball)

2 unpasteurised gherkins, finely chopped

1 teaspoon drained capers, finely chopped

2 tablespoons finely chopped fresh dill

2 tablespoons extra virgin olive oil

Generous pinch mineral-rich salt and black pepper

2 fillets cooked smoked mackerel, approx. 100g each

2 small handfuls watercress

Wash the beetroots and place in a steamer for 45 minutes to 1 hour or until cooked through. Leave to cool and then peel away the skin and chop the beetroots into very small chunks. Add to a small bowl, along with the gherkins, capers and dill. Add the olive oil, salt and pepper and mix well.

Roughly shred the mackerel.

To serve, place a small handful of watercress on each plate and place the mackerel on top. Dot 4 tablespoons of the beet salad around each plate.

tip
Use the leftover salad to pair with poached eggs and sourdough for breakfast the next day.

chicken caesar greens

This is my twist on a classic Caesar salad, using a nut-based dressing that is packed full of flavour and gives the gut a boost. When buying your chicken it is very important to source organic and free range as not only does this have more nutritional value but it also means the animal has been treated fairly – and you really can taste the difference! You can use any leftover dressing for other salads or veggies. If you are vegetarian you can make this dish without the chicken and replace it with a boiled egg. I love this served just as it is but a good slice of sourdough is also a nice accompaniment.

serves 2 (with extra dressing)

2 organic free range chicken breasts, approx. 200g each

Pinch mineral-rich salt and black pepper

1 tablespoon organic unsalted butter or ghee

2 generous handfuls seasonal mixed leaves, washed and patted dry

6–8 caper berries, drained

2 tablespoons shaved Parmesan

caesar dressing

65g cashews, soaked for 2 hours

2 tablespoons pine nuts, soaked for 2 hours

3 tablespoons nutritional yeast flakes

1 tablespoon drained capers

½ teaspoon mustard powder

1 garlic clove, peeled

Juice of ½ lemon

180ml filtered water

Generous pinch mineral-rich salt

First, make the dressing, drain the nuts and rinse thoroughly with filtered water. Place all of the dressing ingredients in a high-speed blender and blend until creamy. Add a little more water if you want a thinner consistency. Transfer to an airtight glass jar and store in the fridge for up to 3 days.

To cook the chicken, you will need a wide shallow pan with a lid. Pound the chicken breasts with a rolling pin to get an even thickness (2–3cm). Season lightly with salt and pepper. Heat the pan, add the butter or ghee and swirl around to coat the pan. Turn the heat to medium and place the chicken breasts in the pan. Cook for 1 minute without moving them. Flip the breasts and then turn the heat to low. Cover with the lid and leave to cook for 10 minutes. Do not lift the lid to check. After the 10 minutes are up, switch off the heat and leave the chicken to rest in the pan for a further 10 minutes. Do not be tempted to lift the lid until the 10 minutes are up! Carefully lift the lid and remove the chicken from the pan.

Place the salad leaves in a large bowl and add the caper berries. Slice the chicken and add to the salad bowl. Stir in 3–4 tablespoons of the Caesar dressing. Top with the Parmesan and enjoy.

green eggs and ham

No prizes for guessing the inspiration behind this recipe. As Dr Seuss's grumpy grouch finds out, he feels great after eating this delectable dish. And indeed this will have your gut and your brain feeling on top of the world. Eggs contain precursors for the production of serotonin, our 'happy hormone'. It's always worth buying organic free range eggs and ham as these generally contain higher levels of omega 3, which is important for regulating anti-inflammatory processes, and that's a good thing for the body overall. Adding my Watercress Pesto provides a hit of this wonderful green veg, which contains plenty of the vitamins and minerals needed for a happier brain–gut connection.

serves 1

2 organic free range eggs

1 tablespoon Watercress Pesto (page 28), plus extra to serve (optional)

1 tablespoon finely chopped fresh basil

Generous pinch mineral-rich salt and black pepper

1 teaspoon organic unsalted butter or ghee

3–4 slices (approx. 125g) organic free range ham

Watercress to garnish (optional)

Crack the eggs into a bowl and whisk. Add the pesto and whisk again to mix evenly. Stir in the basil and seasoning and combine well.

In a frying pan, heat the butter or ghee on a medium heat. Add the egg mix to form an omelette. Cook for 2 minutes on one side and then carefully flip over to cook for 2 minutes on the other side. Transfer to a plate.

Lay the ham on one half of the omelette and flip the other side over to cover. Cut into triangular slices. Add a little extra pinch of salt to finish. If you like, serve with extra Watercress Pesto and garnish with watercress.

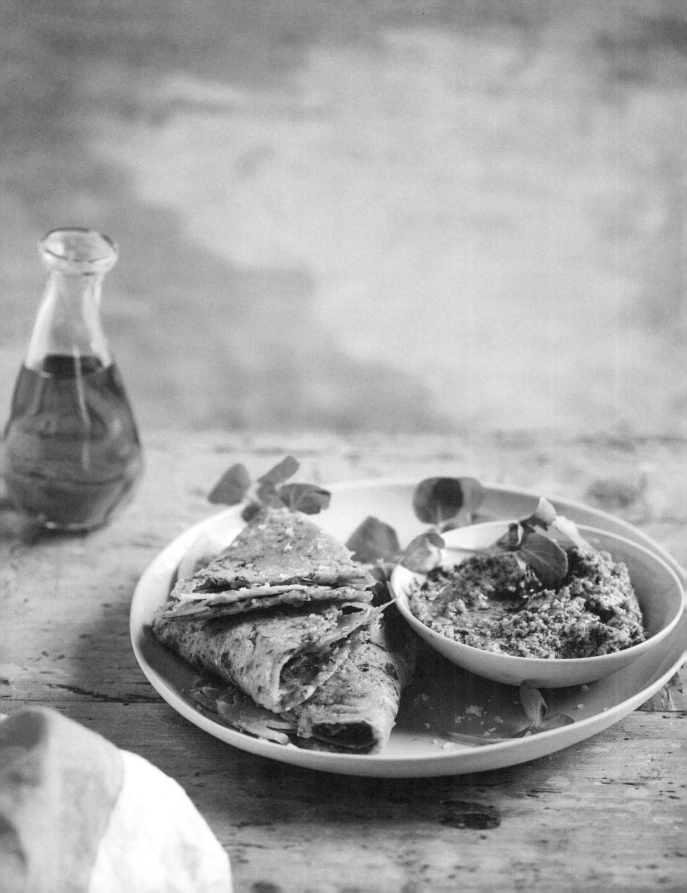

wild salmon with butternut rosemary purée and crispy kale

You could think of this as a scrumptious meeting of mind- and gut-supportive foods. Wild salmon typically boasts a higher level of anti-inflammatory omega 3 essential fatty acids than farmed salmon. Butternut squash can be particularly soothing for the gut and rosemary gives an additional boost for the beneficial bacteria and supports a healthy microbiome. Finish with one of the pin-up foods for healthy eating – kale. This veg supports optimum detoxification and provides nutrients such as B vitamins and magnesium, which are needed for neurotransmitter functioning. It's a dish that will have you thinking and feeling much more relaxed from the first mouthwatering bite!

serves 2

1 butternut squash, peeled and cut into chunks

4 handfuls kale

2 wild salmon fillets, approx. 110g each

Pinch mineral-rich salt and black pepper

1 sprig fresh rosemary

3 tablespoons extra virgin olive oil, plus extra to drizzle

2 tablespoons ghee or organic unsalted butter

Preheat the oven to 200°C/Gas 6. Line two baking trays with baking parchment. Put the chunks of butternut squash on a lined tray and roast for 25–30 minutes until tender.

Meanwhile, prepare the kale by removing the leaves from the stems and cutting into rough chunks.

For the salmon, season lightly with salt and pepper and place on a lined baking tray. Once the butternut squash is cooked, remove from the oven and place the salmon in the oven for 15 minutes.

Transfer the butternut squash into a high-speed blender, then add the rosemary, olive oil and 1 tablespoon of the ghee or butter and generous pinches of salt and pepper. Blend on the highest setting until smooth; you will need to use the tamper to push down the ingredients, or stop and scrape a few times. Transfer to a glass or ceramic container and cover with a plate or lid until you are ready to serve.

Heat the remaining 1 tablespoon of ghee or butter in a shallow pan, add the kale and fry for 3 minutes.

To serve, divide the kale between two plates, add the cooked salmon and 2 generous tablespoons of the butternut purée. Drizzle with a small amount of olive oil and a pinch of mineral-rich salt.

turmeric chicken with laksa zoodles

Laksa sauce has got to be one of the most delicious combinations of flavours and nothing hits the spot like a chicken noodle dish. OK, so the word 'zoodle' might sound gimmicky but it's derived from the American term for courgettes (zucchini) as a play on the word 'noodles'. The point is that these are a fun and easy way to increase your veg intake. The star of this dish, however, is the turmeric used to marinate the chicken: it contains powerful antioxidant and anti-inflammatory compounds that can benefit both the brain and the gut.

serves 2

2 organic free range chicken breasts, approx. 200g each

1 tablespoon organic unsalted butter or ghee

2 teaspoons ground turmeric

2 teaspoons ground cumin

2 generous pinches mineral-rich salt and black pepper

2 courgettes

3 tablespoons desiccated coconut

Small cupped handful cashew nuts, lightly crushed

Handful fresh coriander, roughly chopped

laksa sauce

3 heaped tablespoons unsweetened coconut yogurt

1 teaspoon ground galangal

½ teaspoon ground turmeric

½ teaspoon ground cumin

½ teaspoon ground cinnamon

¼ teaspoon ground cardamom

¼ teaspoon garlic powder

Pinch crushed chilli flakes

Pinch mineral-rich salt

Squeeze fresh lime juice

Preheat the oven to 200°C/Gas 6.

Place the chicken breasts in a bowl and rub with the butter or ghee. Then add the turmeric, cumin, salt and pepper and massage in thoroughly. Wrap each breast in foil to make two parcels and bake for 20–25 minutes until the juices run clear. Remove from the oven and leave to rest for 5–10 minutes.

While the chicken is in the oven, make the zoodles: use a spiraliser to turn the courgettes into 'noodles'. Alternatively, if you don't have a spiraliser, you can grate the courgettes in a food processor or with a box grater. Mix with a pinch of mineral-rich salt and place in a colander. Boil some water and pour over the courgettes to blanch them, then place in a bowl.

To make the laksa sauce, place all the ingredients in a small bowl and mix thoroughly, then add to the zoodles along with the desiccated coconut and stir through.

Slice the chicken across the breast. Divide the dressed zoodles between two plates, top with the sliced chicken and finish with the crushed cashews and chopped coriander.

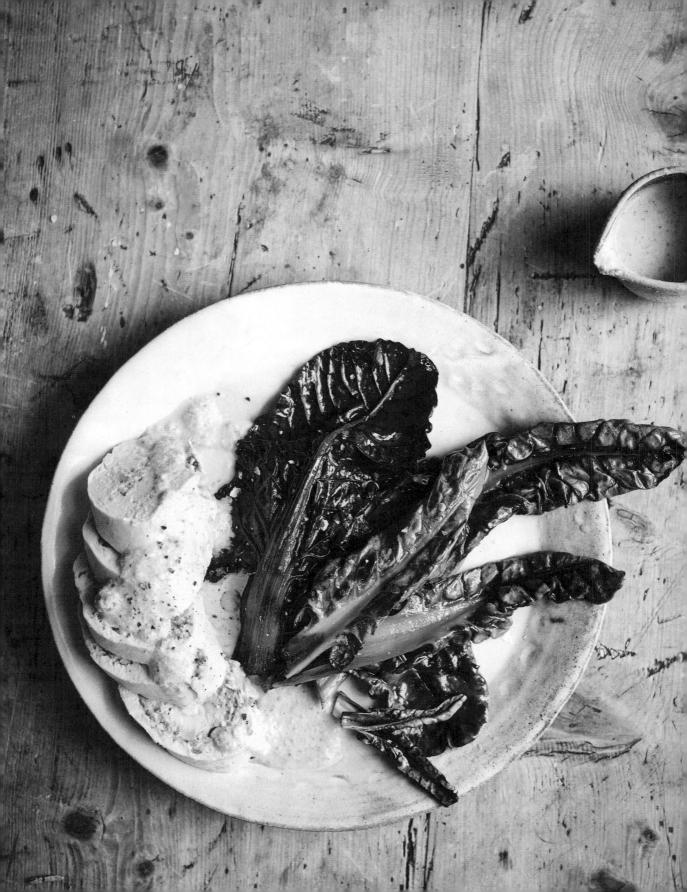

chicken, almond and celery ballotine with wilted chard and creamy caper dressing

This ballotine is deliciously filling and packed full of gut-nourishing foods. Chicken is naturally one of the highest sources of tryptophan, the precursor to serotonin, our 'happy hormone'. I've paired it with wilted chard, as leafy greens are brimming with vitamins and minerals and our gut microbes love the fibre they provide as well. You will have some of the filling left over: pile it into a hot sweet potato or spoon on top of salmon and bake in the oven. Any extra dressing is perfect to perk up fennel or roasted cauliflower; in fact it pretty much works with any vegetables and salads.

serves 2 (with extra filling and dressing)

2 organic free range chicken breasts, approx. 200g each

Organic unsalted butter or ghee

2 handfuls rainbow chard, or other green leafy veg

almond and celery filling

150g almonds with skins, soaked for 8 hours, drained and rinsed with filtered water

2 celery stalks, finely chopped

2 spring onions, finely chopped

1 garlic clove, peeled and finely chopped or crushed

1 tablespoon almond nut butter

¼ teaspoon mild yellow mustard powder

1 tablespoon fresh lemon juice

Generous pinch mineral-rich salt

Pinch black pepper

creamy caper dressing

65g cashews, soaked for 2 hours, drained and rinsed

2 teaspoons drained capers

2 tablespoons nutritional yeast flakes

Pinch mineral-rich salt

Juice of ½ lemon

Place all of the filling ingredients in a food processor and pulse until evenly combined but not too smooth.

Trim any sinews off the chicken breasts. Fold back the fillets so each breast opens out like a book; using a rolling pin, bash them until they are 2–3cm thick. Spread 3 tablespoons of the filling on each of the breasts, fold back the opened side and then roll up tightly. Lightly grease two pieces of foil with a little butter or ghee. Wrap each chicken breast in the foil, making sure to seal the ends to keep in all the juices. Put these in the fridge for 30 minutes.

While the chicken breasts are chilling, make the dressing. Put all of the ingredients into a high-speed blender along with 50ml of filtered water and blend until it has the consistency of double cream; you may need to add more water. Transfer to a sealable glass or ceramic container and place in the fridge. This will keep for up to 3 days.

Preheat the oven to 230°C/Gas 8. Place the chicken parcels on a baking tray and cook for 20 minutes. Remove from the oven and leave to rest for 10 minutes.

While the chicken is resting, trim the rainbow chard stalks if necessary. Heat 1 teaspoon of the butter or ghee in a shallow pan, add the chard and cook for around 5 minutes until wilted.

To serve, cut the chicken into slices about 5cm thick. Divide the chard between two plates, add the chicken and drizzle generously with the caper dressing.

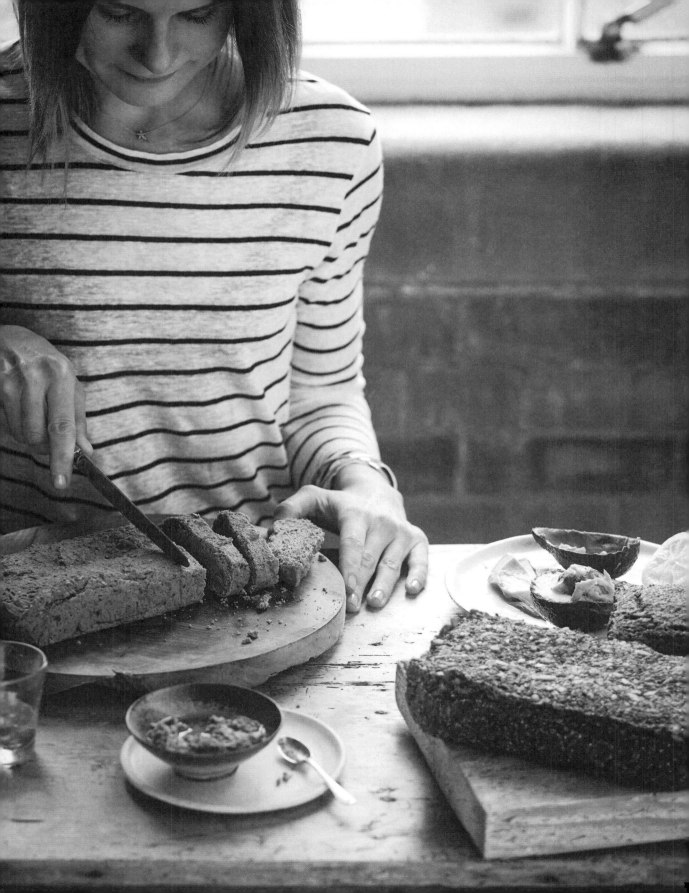

6

what's eating you?

FOOD INTOLERANCES SEEM to be almost the norm these days. How often do you find yourself out for a meal with friends and when it comes to ordering there rises a cacophony of 'I don't eat wheat' or 'Does this have dairy in it?' Before you know it the waiter has to get another note pad just to write down all of the requirements. In supermarkets, the 'free from' aisles are bursting at the seams – and bringing in huge amounts of revenue – as more and more of us look towards these supposedly 'healthier' alternatives. But, given that we have been eating staples such as bread, cheese and milk for millennia, the question is: are these food intolerances genuine, are they just part of a somewhat misguided attempt to follow a healthier lifestyle, or could cutting out certain foods entirely transform a person's health?

In this chapter I aim to uncover the common misconceptions behind some of the most widely avoided foods, and explain why, in shunning some of them, you may be doing yourself, and more specifically your gut, a disservice. I want you to use the knowledge gained from this chapter to make discerning choices about food, rather than blindly cutting out whole food groups without really knowing why. This will allow you to have a healthy and more inclusive diet. I'll also explain the difference between food intolerance and allergy, and how by focusing on specific foods we often miss the underlying point that it is the health of the gut that is most important. Armed with this know-how, you can take a strategic and targeted approach to discovering possible intolerances. If you want to try eliminating certain foods for a period of time to see how you might react – or if you are simply limiting certain foods such as gluten and dairy – you'll find some great alternative recipes in this chapter, including a collection of gloriously creamy nut milks (page 150), a mouthwatering Margherita Cauli Pizza (page 160) and a delicious Super Seed Bread (page 157). They prove that you can lose these kinds of food while keeping the taste factor very much *in* your dishes!

allergy vs intolerance

Some people use the words allergy and intolerance in a very loose way, as if they are somehow interchangeable, but there is a fundamental difference between food allergies and food intolerances.

food allergies

Food allergies create a specific, significant and immediate antigen–antibody response. As we saw in Chapter 4, this means that certain food molecules are perceived by the body to be hostile invaders and the gut responds by producing antibodies (also known as immunoglobulins) to 'fight' the intruders. In the case of allergies, these are IgE antibodies that stimulate certain cells to release histamine, an inflammatory compound. In some cases, this can be life threatening, such as the anaphylactic choking reaction to eating peanuts, caused by a swelling of the tongue or throat. Other food allergy symptoms can include eye and lip swelling, a tightening of the chest and rashes that arise from exposure to any potential allergen. Technically it is possible to have an allergy to *any* food, but the most common allergens include milk, gluten, wheat, nuts, eggs, mustard, sesame, soya and shellfish. For the purposes of this

chapter we'll be focusing on the first two in this group but many of the points will be relevant to any or all allergies.

If you have a food allergy you tend to know about it. It simply isn't possible to have a 'slight allergy' since the symptoms that arise won't be mistakable; they will also be immediately apparent. A blood test will tell you for sure: a food allergy will show up as IgE markers.

Bona fide food allergies are on the increase; in fact by a massive 500 per cent in the last 30 years. They are a very real modern problem. One of the most common is milk allergy, which encompasses all dairy products such as cheese, milk, creams, butter and yogurt. With this allergy the immune system elicits a response to the proteins found in cow's milk, such as casein and whey. In individuals who are susceptible to this allergy, ingesting these proteins will trigger an immediate antibody response that can create extreme reactions of the nature mentioned above.

Another high-profile allergenic food is gluten ('glue' in Latin), which is present in wheat and many cereal grains. It is made up of two proteins, gliadin and glutenin, which give such foods their elastic, sticky, binding character. But the same proteins have catastrophic effects in someone with an allergy to them. This is a diagnosable condition known as coeliac disease, in which the immune system creates antibodies against gluten proteins and mounts an inflammatory 'attacking' autoimmune response against healthy tissue in the gut. Repeated exposure causes damage to the villi in the gut – those guys we met in Chapter 1 that play a fundamental role in the absorption of nutrients. The result is that coeliac sufferers become severely malnourished as they are

Bona fide food allergies are on the increase; in fact by a massive 500 per cent in the last 30 years. They are a very real modern problem.

not able to absorb nutrients from their food, leading to weight loss, fatigue and anaemia. For people with coeliac disease it is paramount that they avoid all products containing gluten, which – along with the disease itself – can be incredibly frustrating and tricky to manage. As well as the usual suspects – breads, pasta, cakes and anything else made with flour – gluten lurks in many sauces, salad dressings, soups and sweets. I guess this is one positive aspect of the 'gluten-free' explosion, since it probably makes shopping and dining out an easier and more pleasurable experience for coeliacs.

Despite the sharp and exponential increase in genuine food allergies, it is estimated they affect only a small percentage of the population. A far greater number of people *'think'* they have an allergy. In most cases they are referring to a food intolerance rather than an allergy.

food intolerances

As we saw above, an allergy is governed by an immediate antigen–IgE antibody immune system response that will show up on a blood test. An intolerance does not involve the immune system in quite the same way and tends to be confined to gut symptoms that are often quite vague in their presentation as well as delayed in onset. Let's explore this in a little bit more detail.

Like allergies, food intolerances can be attributed to various foods, but they can be

much harder to detect and indeed define. In recent years the incidence of intolerances has increased significantly and it is now pretty commonplace for people to say they have some sensitivity to certain foods. But why is that? Some might blame the media or celebrities who have endorsed a gluten- or dairy-free diet that has 'changed their lives' and for sure that needs to be taken into consideration.

Nevertheless, while the immune system won't mount the same extreme response as for an allergy, the physical symptoms of food intolerances can be debilitating for some individuals. Gluten, for example, has been shown to have immediate effects on the gut when ingested by gluten-sensitive non-coeliac individuals: it creates a physical inflammatory reaction even though the sufferer is not medically diagnosed as coeliac. Studies show that non-coeliac gluten sensitivity does exist and although testing via blood is sometimes inconclusive there are inflammatory markers that show an elevation when a sufferer is exposed to gluten-containing foods.

Dairy can also create significant symptoms in the gut. An intolerance to dairy products is generally due to an inability to digest lactose, the natural sugar in dairy, rather than a reaction to the proteins in milk. More accurately referred to as lactose intolerance, this is typically confined to digestive symptoms such as bloating and rapid loose bowel movements, although these can can vary in their presentation and intensity. Some people find that goat and sheep dairy products are better tolerated than cow dairy due to their lower lactose content and shorter amino acid protein chains, which means they are more easily digested.

Testing for food intolerances is usually done via a blood test that measures IgG antibodies related to a delayed inflammatory response, rather than the immediate antigen-related response that occurs with an allergy. However, these tests only provide an indication of foods that may be triggering responses, and sometimes not that accurately, since many of the foods that show up could arguably be more the result of a compromised microbiome and a leaky gut rather than a genuine intolerance to any specific food or food group. Therefore removing suspected triggers from the diet can often be much more demonstrative, at least for the short term, until overall gut health is restored. I'm not suggesting food intolerances don't exist but they are less prevalent than many people think. Certainly if eliminating a food from your diet results in an improvement in symptoms, it is a correlation that cannot be disregarded.

However, before you go 'elimination crazy', it is also important to realise that removing foods from your diet reduces overall variety, which can lead to a limited (and frankly boring) way of eating. Indeed, our modern diet is already narrower than that of our hunter–gatherer ancestors, who consumed a much wider variety of fruits, tubers and vegetables because they had to eat what was available and in season. The consequence of a less diverse diet is a less diverse microbiome and that is detrimental for the gut. With that lack of variety comes over-exposure to the same foods, day in, day out. So, rather than an intolerance, is the problem a system 'overload' due to repeated exposure to the same foods? Let's take gluten as an example. It isn't unusual for many of us to have cereal at breakfast, a sandwich at lunch and pasta in the evening, and while on the face of it that may sound like a fairly nutritious day, particularly if all the carbs are wholemeal, it means exposure to gluten at every single meal. Perhaps the phrase too much of a good thing might be more appropriate than thinking in terms of intolerance.

We also need to take into consideration the other ingredients that are included in a lot of our foods, such as artificial sweeteners, preservatives, emulsifiers, hydrogenated fats and pesticide residues. These substances can contribute to, and indeed cause, an inflammatory response. So gluten or dairy may not be the cause after all. This is something we cannot ignore and it is highly relevant if we are to avoid the vilification of perfectly healthy foods. Additives and other chemicals can elicit gut symptoms all by themselves, so rather than avoiding entire food groups perhaps you should think more about eating foods in their most natural state. The point is that in our attempt to remove all these 'bad' foods and follow the illustrious concept of 'clean eating' we are further restricting our diet, and that has its own ramifications, particularly when it comes to the gut and our microbiome.

feed your microbes

It is crucial to understand that when we think about reactions to foods we also need to consider the trillions of microbes in the gut and the intestinal barrier.

I often see clients who tried to manage their symptoms by cutting out a whole food group; they may find a bit of relief initially but then the symptoms return so they cut out another, and so on. Eventually they end up with a very narrow and frankly nutritionally depleted diet while still suffering with the same issues. That's because removing foods can be irrelevant if there are fundamental imbalances in the gut that are driving gut-related symptoms in the first place.

Before we can pinpoint potential trigger foods we first need to support the microbiome. Bacterial imbalances in the gut can create symptoms irrespective of what you are eating. If you think back to the leaky gut scenario discussed in Chapter 4, you'll remember that dysbiosis can damage the gut lining, resulting in it becoming more permeable. This can potentially allow various food proteins into the bloodstream, creating an inflammatory reaction that may be mistaken for a food intolerance response, which means that leaky gut in itself can create reactions to foods. So rather than randomly cutting out foods, we really need to think about supporting the microbiome and the integrity of the gut barrier. Using the Weed, Seed and Feed programme (page 46) can help you to do just that and guide you through how to strategically remove certain foods. Once the gut has found its equilibrium and is more robust, it is often the case that those foods that may previously have created a reaction no longer have the same effect.

Indeed some vilified food groups, such as gluten and dairy, actually provide support for the gut, as long as a little caution is exercised in the types that are chosen and they are eaten in moderation. Bread and milk should not necessarily be seen as 'bad' and removed without a second thought; the way they have been prepared or processed can make all the difference. For example, in Chapter 4 we looked at 'anti-nutrient' compounds in grains: these compounds can be minimised through soaking and sprouting, and therefore don't create the same symptoms as the refined

types. Similarly, milk and cheese made in the traditional way provide us with bountiful nutrition and tons of beneficial microbes. Let's look at this more closely, starting with one of the most stigmatised of all foods – bread.

why bread isn't all bad

Poor bread. When it comes to nutrition, it has had a bad rap in recent decades. The low carb diet obsession didn't help, and bread is also often called out for its ability to make people bloated and put on weight. But is that really the case? For millennia, all bread was leavened using naturally occurring yeasts. However, after the introduction of commercial yeasts, bread became more widely available, but it was also more manipulated and tasteless, with a long list of additives and other suspect ingredients. The majority of bread today is prepared and processed in a completely different way from its naturally fermented ancestor – sourdough.

Sourdough is made with minimal ingredients and like other fermented foods uses a starter culture that allows bacteria to flourish. In the case of sourdough this is a mix of flour and water that is left in a warm place to ferment and multiply. As its name suggests, sourdough has a distinctive sour taste that comes from the airborne wild yeasts and *Lactobacilli* bacteria that develop in the starter: the slightly 'off' smell is the result of those bacteria and the acids produced during fermentation simply 'doing their thing'. Once the starter is good to go you can make your sourdough. It is the long fermentation process that makes sourdough generally much more digestible than other types of bread, as the lactic and acetic acids work to predigest starches in the grains. These same acids also help to neutralise phytates, some of the chemical 'anti-nutrient' substances mentioned in Chapter 4. These occur naturally in grains and can create digestive discomfort as well as affecting the absorption of nutrients that sourdough has to offer, which include iron, zinc, magnesium and folic acid.

Furthermore, because of this fermentation process, the gluten in the flour is almost entirely degraded into amino acids so it becomes easier to digest and less likely to cause reactions. This has been demonstrated in studies where individuals who usually react to gluten showed normal values of blood and intestinal markers when consuming fresh sourdough.

All of this goes to highlight the fact that even where food allergies or intolerances are concerned it is a lot more complicated than simply ruling out food groups that can have lots of nutritional benefits. This leads us nicely on to the other big debate: dairy.

the dairy dilemma

'Little Miss Muffet sat on a tuffet, eating her curds and whey' – unless she had a problem with dairy! Like bread, dairy hasn't had it easy PR-wise in recent years. It started with the outcry about the fat content, especially saturated fat, which we have now realised is largely nonsense. The demonisation of dairy fat led many people to opt for 'healthy' margarine alternatives to butter, which, it turns out, are often laced with far more damaging synthetic trans fats, rather than the healthy saturated fats that you find in butter. Then came the upsurge of lactose intolerance, with many people declaring themselves 'off dairy' for many different and sometimes absurd reasons.

Whatever your opinion of dairy, most conventional nutritionists would recognise it as a valuable food source that is rich in protein and calcium and provides vitamins A, D and K_2, the latter of which is otherwise hard to find in the diet. Moreover, full fat dairy also contains compounds such as butyrate and conjugated linoleic acid (CLA) that both have beneficial effects. Butyrate, as mentioned in Chapter 2, provides energy for the colon cells, helps manage inflammation and has a protective role in the gut. CLA is a natural trans fat that has been positively linked with reducing the risk of heart disease and diabetes.

However, some people do argue that dairy isn't healthy for human consumption. There are a couple of reasons for this. The first is that, after we have been weaned, we fail to produce lactase, the enzyme needed to break down the sugar in milk (lactose). (Breast milk is loaded with lactose that most of us can tolerate and forms a complete food source for us to grow.) However, this argument fails to acknowledge the role of evolution. When humans started consuming cow's milk, some 10,000 years ago, a genetic process called 'lactase persistence' meant that our genes mutated to continue the production of lactase into adulthood so that we could break down lactose effectively. This was in the interests of our survival and reproduction, and the success of the process is evident in the fact that close to 99 per cent of all northern Europeans nowadays have the necessary genes to digest lactose.

The other assertion is that we humans shouldn't drink milk because no other mammal drinks another mammal's milk. Well, there are a lot of things we do with our food that other animals don't, like cooking it for a start, so that argument doesn't really stand up either. Nevertheless, there are many people who suffer with debilitating gut symptoms after eating dairy, so why are they suddenly having all these problems?

Let's take a look at what has happened to our food in the last few decades, using milk as a prime example. Like many of my generation, sipping from a small bottle of creamy full fat milk is one of my fondest childhood memories, and growing up in the sticks in Wales it usually came from freely roaming cows on our local farm. But that milk was a very far cry from much of what currently graces the shelves of our supermarkets. The white liquid masquerading as milk can be an entirely different end product from how it started.

These days, milk in the supermarket is always sold pasteurised, which is a method of heat-treatment used to kill potentially pathogenic bacteria. Pasteurisation was invented over a century ago as a life saving and necessary measure to avoid contamination by harmful bacteria. Back then they didn't have the same hygiene, sanitation or refrigeration that we do now. However, this indiscriminate killing process also eradicates the beneficial microbes, and, in case you hadn't already gathered, these guys are pretty important for our health. Pasteurisation also destroys natural enzymes present in the milk that help us to digest and absorb it properly; crucially these include lactase, which as mentioned above is needed to break down lactose. This begs the question of whether people are actually lactose intolerant or if the milk they are drinking simply lacks some of its natural supporting co-factors.

The other technique used in standard milk production is homogenisation, a high-pressure process to break down the fat into smaller components. This creates a uniform consistency so that the milk looks more 'attractive' and the cream doesn't sit at the top. However, the process oxidises fats and as such creates free radicals – molecules that can cause inflammation in the body. Not so pretty. Some argue that this reconfiguration of particles also has implications for the gut and digestion.

Then we have fat-reduced milks, in which the crucial 'fat' factor needed for the fat-soluble vitamins to be absorbed is missing. This means that those nutrients need to be added back in. Some low-fat milk substitutes also contain thickening agents. Can we really call it milk after all of that? Frankly it's no wonder the gut has problems digesting it. For most of us, that's got little to do with lactose intolerance and more to do with the removal of all the crucial components that make milk ... well, milk.

what to choose from the dairy

Let's backtrack a bit here, all the way to 400BC. Hippocrates, known as the father of medicine, supposedly used dairy liberally, in its natural and cultured forms, when treating his patients. He was also a champion of the gut, having famously written 'all disease begins in the gut', and he made the connection between these natural cultured sources of probiotics and the positive effects they had on digestion. Indeed if you go back to before modern processing methods and look at milk and dairy in its most natural state one could argue that it is a very different product. Raw dairy milk, because it is unpasteurised, contains all of its natural enzymes and beneficial bacteria, which contribute to the health of the gut and

kefir

Kefir is a fermented milk beverage that has been revered in Eastern Europe, Russia and Central Asia for centuries. Tart to taste and a game changer in its nutritional rewards, this effervescent, sour milk drink contains a ton of beneficial bacteria and yeasts. Like many fermented foods, it needs some kind of starter that allows the bacteria to flourish and with kefir this comes in the form of 'grains', which look like wobbly mini cauliflower florets. Yes they look a bit weird, but these alien-like blobs are home to more than twenty beneficial microorganisms that make kefir one of the most microbial-rich foods around. As you continue to 'feed' the grains they grow and multiply and then you can pass some on to your nearest and dearest so they can start their own culturing process. Regular feeding is required for them to thrive – just like a pet – so for most of us, draining and drinking the kefir and then feeding the grains can form part of a morning microbial ritual. The bountiful supply of bacteria in kefir is one of the major reasons why it has long been revered for its effects in supporting the gut and microbiome.

The other great thing about kefir is that because of the way it is fermented the lactose content is reduced to around 1 per cent and those who usually suffer from lactose intolerance find that drinking it regularly actually improves their digestion, rather than creating the unpleasant symptoms they normally experience when drinking milk. It is undoubtedly one of nature's best natural probiotics and one that has stood the test of time. Check out my recipe on page 153 so you can start to culture your own.

the immune system. However, the decision to drink raw milk has to be a personal one, as opinions are divided on the matter. But the fact is that farmers producing raw milk still need to adhere to specific controls. All things considered, the taste and health benefits make it my preferred option. To buy raw milk, you need to go to farmers that produce it (see page 264). The process of fermentation in other cultured dairy products may also provide similar health benefits. Yogurt is probably the most renowned for its health properties. Sadly, many of the yogurts we can buy are processed in the same ways as milk, so try to buy full fat natural organic or the sheep or goat versions, as these tend to be closer to the real deal.

cheese

The American writer Clifton Fadiman described cheese as 'milk's leap toward immortality', and it is one of my personal dairy delights. Beyond that stinky exterior you'll find a host of nutritional benefits that our gut microbes love. Cheese-making has been around for some 9000 years and for the vast majority of those it was practised as an artisanal craft. The mass production of rennet changed that, as it meant cheese could be made on a much bigger scale, but that means some supermarket variations are very different from their traditional ancestors.

Fortunately for you and your gut, cheese has seen a renaissance, with smaller farm-based producers offering exceptional and tasty varieties. Incredible flavour aside, these types of cheese are a nutritionally superior and wholly healthy addition to our diet.

Fortunately for you and your gut, cheese has seen a renaissance, with smaller farm-based producers offering exceptional and tasty varieties. Incredible flavour aside, these types of cheese can be a wholly healthy addition to our diet and can have a positive influence on our gut too. And this is where it gets interesting from a health perspective. We know that cheese is high in fat, but the saturated fats it contains, when eaten in moderation, have been linked to the prevention of certain chronic diseases and help our microbiome to support anti-inflammatory processes. Many traditionally made cheeses are a great source of probiotics due to the fermentation process they undergo. However, cheeses that are made from unpasteurised (raw) milk are more likely to provide a greater quantity and diversity of beneficial bacteria than their pasteurised counterparts, making them more supportive for the microbiome. They taste better too!

So be discerning with your cheese buying. Squeezy, rubbery slices don't count: separating good quality cheese from the processed stuff is the main thing. Farmers' markets are great but in a supermarket a glance at the label will confirm if a cheese is unpasteurised: those are the cheeses that give the maximum nutritional benefits. Always go for full fat and choose organic where possible, as these include omega 3 essential fatty acids that support anti-inflammatory processes. Check out my Celeriac and Kraut Rösti with

Poached Eggs and Halloumi (page 248) or the beautiful Beetroot and Goats' Cheese Stacks (page 30) for some cheesy inspiration.

your diy elimination diet

So we have looked at allergies, intolerances and some of the main 'culprit' foods but it is important to realise that ultimately we are all individuals. Just as we laugh at different things and have various tastes in movies, your body won't work the same as the next person's either. So we have to tune in to ourselves to understand whether certain foods are causing a problem. It might be tempting to invest in an IgG food intolerance test to see which foods don't sit well with you, but if you have a gut that is out of balance these tests can show false negatives and positives as I mentioned earlier.

Start with supporting your gut. If you want a true picture of the foods that may be causing symptoms then full elimination of the potential triggers is the most accurate measure. That means taking a specific food group out of the diet entirely for a minimum of six weeks and then reintroducing one of the foods every three days, without any other 'new' food on the days that you are reintroducing them, so any reaction is not open to misinterpretation. That might mean having natural, unsweetened cow's milk yogurt one day and then not having any other eliminated food for another three days. It is important to follow this timing as it can take a few days for symptoms to manifest. You'll soon realise if you are reacting to certain foods and it may be a question of not eating them for now and then maybe trying again in a month or two. That's why supporting the gut on a much deeper level needs to be part of this strategy. My Weed, Seed and Feed programme on page 46 can give you a good head start.

There is a misconception that 'free from' products are healthier than their gluten and dairy containing counterparts, which very often simply isn't the case.

When choosing alternatives to dairy and gluten during the elimination period, remember the mantra of eating foods in their most natural state and avoid the supermarket 'free from' aisles. There is a misconception that 'free from' products are healthier than their gluten- and dairy-containing counterparts, which very often simply isn't the case. For example, if you're swapping dairy milk for plant-based 'milk', then ideally make your own from scratch (you'll find my nut milk recipes on page 150 very useful). If you are buying it then check it doesn't contain unnecessary fillers: almond milk should have almonds, water and perhaps a bit of salt and that's it. If you're avoiding gluten, try some of my delicious breads like the Super Seed Bread

(page 157) or Cinnamon Loaf (page 224) or just eat soaked or sprouted grains in their original form. There are plenty of tasty and easy recipes in the book so you can make your own gluten- and grain-free dishes. That way you will know that they are made from whole ingredients.

be inclusive not exclusive

You will have learnt over the last few pages that the way in which we respond to foods goes beyond the food itself and crucially is governed by the health of the gut and the microbiome. Hopefully, having read this chapter and looked back to the Weed, Seed and Feed programme you now have an understanding of how to eliminate possible trigger foods using a strategic and targeted approach that fundamentally supports and rebalances the gut. The important point is that the aim, in the long term, is to be 'inclusive' and enjoy a wide variety of foods. That approach – rather than removing foods from the diet haphazardly – is often the best way to support the gut. Eating the same foods over and over, whether 'healthy' or not, isn't the goal here.

Diversity and rotation are important. Our microbes like, and in fact need, diversity in what we eat to maintain diversity in their numbers and species. Mixing it up and varying the menu keeps the microbiome hungry for a wide variety of foods and creates a happy gut. Rather than eliminating an entire food group it's important to be more discerning about the foods themselves, to avoid missing out on some crucial nutrients and natural probiotics. When it comes to being good to your gut, it seems inclusive is the new 'free from'!

gingerbread granola

Spicy gingerbread has got to be one of the ultimate treats and in this granola form it's also great for your gut. This recipe is based on sprouted oats and activated nuts (see page 16) that make them more easily digested than their raw form and also makes for better nutrient absorption. Those famous spices that make up this classic biscuit and a touch of maca powder, which gives additional flavour and a nutritional boost, mean this moorish granola will certainly put a spring in your morning step. I think it's delicious served with raw dairy milk but it also works brilliantly with Cashew Milk (page 151).

serves 8–10

150g activated almonds

125g activated pecans

100g activated walnuts

100g sprouted oats

3 tablespoons ground flaxseed (ideally sprouted – see page 264)

2 teaspoons ground ginger

1 teaspoon cinnamon

½ teaspoon ground cloves

1 teaspoon ground allspice

½ teaspoon ground nutmeg

Seeds from 1 vanilla pod

1 tablespoon maca powder

Pinch black pepper

Generous pinch mineral-rich salt

3 tablespoons raw honey, melted (use coconut nectar blossom for a vegan version)

1 tablespoon melted organic unsalted butter or ghee (use coconut oil for a vegan version)

Preheat the oven to 150°C/Gas 2. Line baking sheet with parchment paper.

Place the nuts into a food processor and pulse a few times to break down a bit into smaller chunks. Transfer into a large bowl. Add the oats, ground flaxseed, spices, vanilla, maca and salt and pepper. Stir thoroughly.

Add the melted honey and butter and mix thoroughly until well coated. Transfer onto the baking tray and bake for 20 minutes. Stir around and place back into the oven for a further 10 minutes.

Allow to cool and store in an airtight glass or ceramic container for up to 1 month.

the milks

I've pulled together a collection of my favourite nut milk recipes for those who are following a plant-based diet, react badly to lactose or just want to mix it up with regular dairy milk. They will also help you to avoid commercial dairy milk during the Weed, Seed and Feed programme. What's more, these nut versions have their own unique nutritional properties. For example Brazil nuts are considered to be one of the best sources of selenium, an important antioxidant that is essential for the function of the thyroid, while cashews are an excellent source of copper, needed by the body to support energy production. Hazelnuts contain high levels of polyphenols, which is great news for the gut as these help to support the growth of beneficial microbes. Use these milks just as you would regular milk. I think cashew is best in tea and coffee but they all work superbly in bircher muesli, such as my blueberry version (page 102), or with Hazelnut, Cardamom and Cacao Granola (page 174) or in the smoothie bowl recipes (pages 55 and 127). One thing you do need is a nut milk bag – but an old pair of tights does the trick.

brazil nut milk

makes 1 litre

140g Brazil nuts, soaked for 4 hours, drained and rinsed with filtered water
Seeds from 1 vanilla pod or 3 drops vanilla extract
Pinch mineral-rich salt

Blend the Brazil nuts and 1 litre of filtered water in a high-speed blender. Once fully blended, strain through a nut milk bag into a large jug; this will take 3–5 minutes.

Pour the milk back into the blender and blend with the vanilla and salt. Transfer the milk into a glass bottle and store in the fridge for up to 3 days.

cashew milk

125g cashews, soaked for
2 hours, drained and rinsed
with filtered water

Seeds from 1 vanilla pod or
3 drops vanilla extract

Pinch mineral-rich salt

Put all of the ingredients into a high-speed blender with
1 litre of filtered water and pulse until blended into a creamy
milk texture. If you have a powerful enough blender, cashew
milk usually doesn't require straining through a nut milk
bag, but if it does contain small pieces then you can do that
now. Pour into a glass bottle and store in the fridge for up to
3 days.

hazelnut milk

makes 1 litre

130g hazelnuts, soaked for
8 hours, drained and rinsed
with filtered water

Seeds from 1 vanilla pod or
3 drops vanilla extract

Pinch mineral-rich salt

Blend the hazelnuts and 1 litre of filtered water in a high-
speed blender. Once fully blended, strain through a nut milk
bag into a large jug.

Pour the milk back into the blender and blend with the
vanilla and salt. Transfer the milk into a glass bottle and store
in the fridge for up to 3 days.

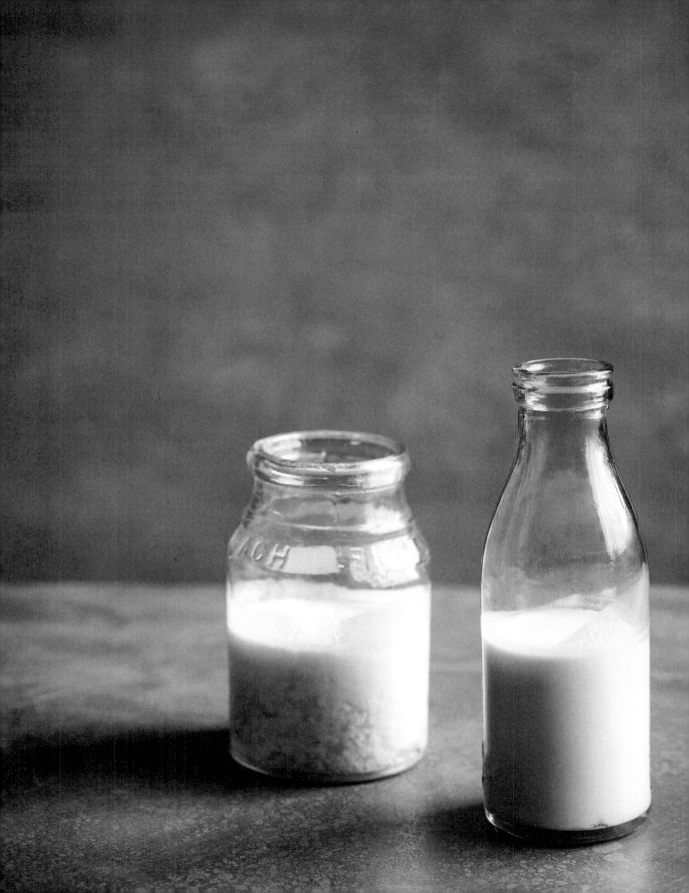

kefir

Where do I start with the benefits of kefir? Firstly, what is it exactly? Well, it's a refreshing, slightly fizzy fermented milk drink that has a tart taste similar to yogurt and it contains multiple strains of bacteria and beneficial yeasts, making it a rich and diverse source of natural probiotics. Because of this it has been linked to improving general digestive health as well as gut-related conditions. And it is delicious, although it may take a while to get used to the taste. Don't be put off by the weird 'grains' that you need to ferment the milk; these guys are making something pretty special, after all (my shopping guide on page 262 tells you where to get these grains). My personal preference is for raw (unpasteurised and unhomogenised) dairy milk, but if that's not available then organic unhomogenised full fat milk is the next best option. The optimal time to drink your kefir is first thing in the morning as it gets you into a good routine, and you can add it to smoothies or serve with other dishes as suggested throughout the book. I've also included two options for coconut kefir.

dairy kefir
2 tablespoons live milk kefir grains

500ml raw or organic unhomogenised full fat milk

coconut kefir
option 1
(needs to be reactivated with dairy milk every few batches to keep the grains strong)

2 tablespoons live milk kefir grains

500ml full fat coconut milk

option 2
3 tablespoons live water kefir grains

500ml full fat coconut milk

In a clean glass jar add the kefir grains and top with the milk. Cover with a muslin cloth and leave in a warm place to ferment. The dairy version will take around 24 hours, coconut around 12 hours.

After this time, use a plastic strainer and a wooden spoon to strain the liquid into a ceramic bowl, keeping the grains in the strainer. It is important not to use a metal spoon or strainer as this can affect the bacteria. Transfer the strained kefir into a glass bottle and store what you don't drink immediatly in the fridge. Rinse the glass jar clean using filtered water and spoon the grains back in. Top up again with milk. Repeat this process every day.

If you are making coconut kefir using option 1, then every three batches use dairy milk for 24 hours to revitalise the grains.

If you decide to have a break or go on holiday, top up the grains with milk and store in the fridge for up to 7 days. For longer periods – up to 14 days – place the grains in a glass without milk in the fridge.

tip
Kefir will keep in the fridge for up to 3 days.

tofu coconut-crumbed dippers with satay sauce

These dippers are a fun, delicious vegan dish that's great for the gut. And kids love them too. I have used a 'breadcrumb' mix of cashews, peanut butter and desiccated coconut to give a sweet taste and crispy texture that go brilliantly with the easy satay sauce. This works well with pea shoots or a green leafy salad and sliced avocado; alternatively, Wasabi Broccoli (page 34) is a nice side. It is important to source your tofu well, making sure it is made from organic and non-genetically modified soya beans and with no added ingredients. I have given some suggestions on where to buy the best on page 265.

serves 2

280–325g non-GMO organic plain tofu

65g activated cashews (page 16)

20g desiccated coconut

1 teaspoon unsweetened peanut butter

Pinch mineral-rich salt

150g coconut flour

6 tablespoons coconut aminos

satay sauce

1 tablespoon unsweetened peanut butter

1 tablespoon unsweetened coconut yogurt

¼ teaspoon garlic powder

1 tablespoon coconut aminos (or you can substitute tamari)

Preheat the oven to 200°C/Gas 6 and line a baking tray with baking parchment.

Prepare the tofu by patting dry and cutting in half lengthwise. Then cut each half into three and finally cut each of these sections in half diagonally, making 12 triangles in total.

To make the coconut crumb, put the cashews, coconut, peanut butter and a pinch of salt into a food processor and pulse until you get fine, even crumbs. Put this mixture to one side.

Next, prepare your dipping stations. Put 6 tablespoons of coconut flour on a large plate. Put the coconut aminos in a bowl. On another large plate, put 6 tablespoons of coconut flour and 6 tablespoons of the coconut crumb and stir to combine evenly. Put your tofu pieces through the dipping stations: first into the straight coconut flour to coat evenly, then into the aminos, turning to get all of the tofu covered, and finally into the coconut crumb mix, making sure that the pieces are thoroughly coated. Place them on the baking tray. Bake for 20 minutes and then turn carefully and return to the oven for a further 10 minutes.

While the tofu is cooking, mix together all of the ingredients for the satay sauce in a small bowl. Divide the tofu dippers between two plates and serve with the sauce.

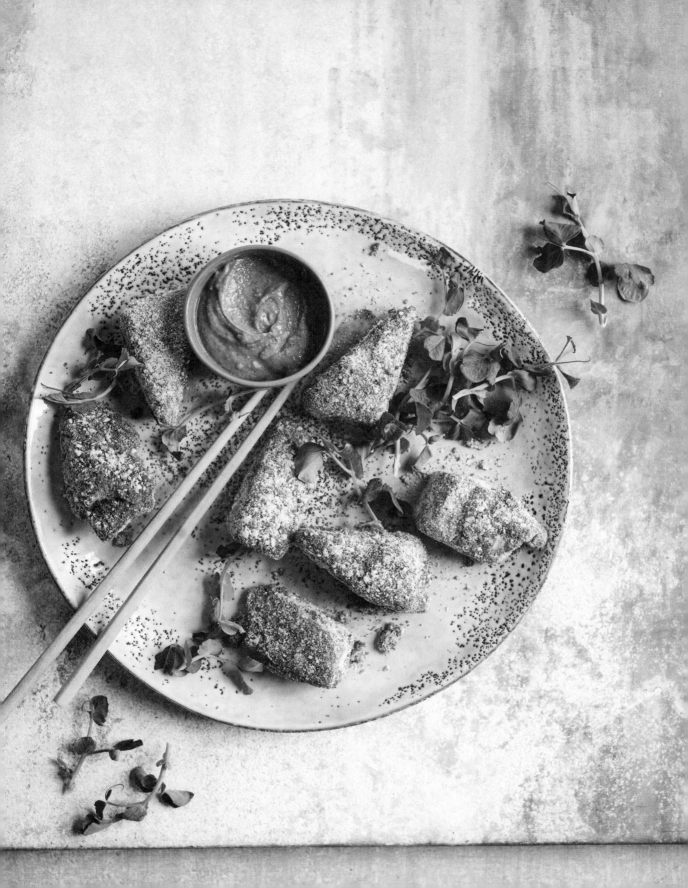

pea and broad bean parsnip 'risotto'

This take on a classic risotto is enhanced by the flavour of parsnip, which also provides a beneficial boost of fibre for the microbes in the gut. As an added bonus, the parsnip version is much quicker and easier to make than regular risotto. It's a surprisingly filling dish but some buttery wilted spinach on the side is a welcome addition. Oh, and a nice chilled glass of biodynamic white wine (see page 261).

serves 2

50g garden peas

50g broad beans

½ tablespoon organic unsalted butter or ghee (use coconut oil for a vegan version)

2 garlic cloves, peeled and finely chopped or crushed

2 tablespoons fresh thyme leaves

1 tablespoon apple cider vinegar

parsnip 'rice'

2 parsnips, peeled and roughly chopped

½ teaspoon garlic powder

½ teaspoon onion powder

3 tablespoons extra virgin olive oil

2 tablespoons nutritional yeast flakes

Pinch mineral-rich salt and plenty of cracked black pepper

to serve

Extra virgin olive oil to drizzle

Grated Parmesan (omit for a vegan version)

Couple of sprigs fresh thyme

Cook the peas and broad beans, then put to one side.

To make the parsnip rice, put the chopped parsnips in a food processor and pulse until you have small pieces. Add all of the other rice ingredients and process until you have a rice-like texture. Place in a small bowl to one side.

Melt the butter or ghee in a medium–large saucepan, add the peas, beans, garlic, thyme and vinegar and cook for 2–3 minutes. Then add the parsnip rice and cook for a few minutes until fully heated through.

Divide between two plates. Drizzle with the olive oil, top with the Parmesan and a pinch of mineral-rich salt and garnish with the thyme.

super seed bread

This loaf is deeply nourishing and satisfying; a little goes a long way as it has a dense texture similar to that of traditional rye or pumpernickel bread (you can see it on the right in the photo on page 138). It's based on nuts and seeds, which are excellent sources of fibre and polyphenols, while the addition of parsnip and carrot not only boosts the fibre content but also gives a flavoursome kick. Psyllium husks are also renowned for getting the gut moving along nicely.

It keeps for up to a week, so it's perfect for lunch or when you get home in the evening. I love it with some smoked salmon and sliced avocado as an open sandwich, or it goes really well alongside my Spicy Parsnip Satay Soup (page 83).

makes 1 loaf

2 tablespoons psyllium husks powder

360ml filtered water

1 medium parsnip (approx. 150g), peeled

1 medium carrot (approx. 135g), peeled

150g activated almonds with skins (page 16)

65g activated sunflower seeds (page 16)

60g activated pumpkin seeds (page 16)

55g sesame seeds

75g chia seeds

1 teaspoon caraway seeds

1 teaspoon cumin seeds

2 tablespoons melted ghee or organic unsalted butter (use coconut oil for a vegan version)

1 teaspoon mineral-rich salt

Mix the psyllium husks powder with the water in a small bowl until it forms a gel (5–10 minutes).

Meanwhile, shred the parsnip and carrot in a food processor, then transfer to a large bowl and place to one side. Rinse and dry the food processor.

Put the almonds and all the seeds into the food processor and pulse very briefly until roughly chopped. Add to the bowl with the parsnip and carrot, then add the melted ghee or butter, salt and psyllium gel and stir well to combine fully. Set aside for 1 hour.

Preheat the oven to 180°C/Gas 4. Grease a 23 x 12cm loaf tin. Spoon the mixture into the tin and level the top. Bake for 1 hour, then check that it's done by turning out and tapping the bottom: it should sound hollow. If not, return it to the oven for 5–10 minutes. Turn out on to a wire rack and leave to cool completely before slicing.

sticky bbq tempeh with five-spice turnip 'rice'

I love this take on sticky barbecued ribs. Tempeh is made from fermented soya beans and because of the fermentation process it is one of the most gut-friendly foods you can eat. In this recipe it is baked with a sweet sticky marinade that is so tasty you'll be making it all the time and using it in other dishes – I love it on Happy Cow Burgers (page 180). The great thing is that unlike a lot of shop-bought barbecue sauces, which typically contain a load of refined sugar, the sweetness and stickiness come from raw honey, which has its own gut-boosting benefits. Piled on top of egg-fried turnip 'rice' that contains bountiful prebiotics, this is lip-smackingly good.

serves 2

200g non-GMO tempeh

2 heads pak choi

1 tablespoon coconut oil

1 tablespoon coconut aminos

Coriander leaves and sesame seeds to garnish

Sesame oil to drizzle

sticky marinade

3 tablespoons tomato paste

2 teaspoons raw honey (use date syrup for a vegan version)

½ tablespoon apple cider vinegar

2 tablespoons coconut aminos

1 teaspoon ground cumin

½ teaspoon garlic powder

1 teaspoon onion powder

1 teaspoon smoked mild paprika

¼ teaspoon mustard powder

½ teaspoon ground cinnamon

Pinch chipotle chilli flakes or regular chilli flakes

Generous pinch mineral-rich salt and black pepper

turnip 'rice'

1 medium turnip (approx. 120g), peeled and cut into rough chunks

1 teaspoon Chinese five spice powder

7–9 very fine red chilli slices (add more or less depending on how spicy you want it)

2 spring onions, finely sliced

Pinch mineral-rich salt

1 tablespoon coconut oil

1 organic free range egg (omit for a vegan version)

Preheat the oven to 180°C/Gas 4 and line a baking tray with baking parchment. Mix the marinade ingredients in a small bowl. Cut the tempeh into six slices. Coat each slice evenly with the marinade and place on the lined tray. Bake for 20 minutes.

While the tempeh is cooking, make the turnip rice. Put the turnip into a food processor and pulse until you have a rice-like texture. Transfer to a bowl and add the five spice, chilli, spring onions and salt.

To cook the rice, heat the coconut oil in a saucepan on a medium heat, add the rice and stir-fry for 4 minutes. Crack in the egg and fry for a further 2 minutes, stirring constantly to break up the egg through the rice.

Trim the ends of the pak choi. Heat some coconut oil in a frying pan, add the pak choi and stir-fry for 2 minutes, then add the coconut aminos.

To serve, divide the turnip rice between two plates, add the pak choi on top and rest the sticky tempeh slices on the side. Garnish with fresh coriander, sesame seeds and a drizzle of sesame oil.

tip

If turnips don't flick your switch you can always use quinoa, as it works wonderfully with the five-spiced blend, or another veg such as cauliflower or parsnip.

margherita cauli pizza

I created this for a vegan friend of mine who was diagnosed coeliac and desperately missed pizza. Entirely unimpressed by a lot of the gluten-free versions, I'm happy to report that she gave this recipe a resounding thumbs up from a taste and a digestion point of view! The recipe doesn't have a flour base and instead uses cauliflower and ground almonds, which give a really lovely, almost crunchy, texture. This uses a cashew cheese, but if you are not vegan you can use unpasteurised Manchego instead as that works superbly for the gut too. Best served with a green leafy salad that includes fresh mint and some seeds, with a decent drizzle of extra virgin olive oil.

serves 4

½ medium–large cauliflower, cut roughly into florets

3 tablespoons ground flaxseed

50g ground almonds

½ teaspoon dried oregano

¼ teaspoon garlic powder

¼ teaspoon mineral-rich salt

cashew cheese

65g cashews, soaked for 2 hours, drained and rinsed

4 tablespoons nutritional yeast flakes

Generous pinch mineral-rich salt

Juice of ½ lemon

120ml filtered water

topping

1 tablespoon ghee or organic unsalted butter

1 red onion, peeled and thinly sliced

10–12 cherry tomatoes, sliced in half

1 garlic clove, peeled and crushed

Basil leaves, roughly torn

Preheat the oven to 200°C/Gas 6 and line a baking sheet with baking parchment.

Place the cauliflower florets in a food processor and pulse until you have a fine rice-like texture.

In a large bowl, mix the ground flaxseed with 6 tablespoons of filtered water to get a sticky texture. Add the almonds, oregano, garlic powder and salt, along with the cauliflower, and use your hands to mix together and create a 'dough'. Spread this on the baking sheet to form a circle about 5mm thick and place in the oven for 45 minutes. Remove from the oven and set aside to cool and crisp.

To make the cashew cheese, place all the ingredients in a food processor and blend until you have a smoothish texture.

To make the topping, heat the ghee or butter in a frying pan and sauté the onion until soft. Add the tomatoes and then the garlic and cook for a further 2 minutes. Remove from the heat and stir through the basil leaves.

To assemble, spread the cashew cheese over the pizza base and then add the tomato topping. Finish with a generous pinch of mineral-rich salt.

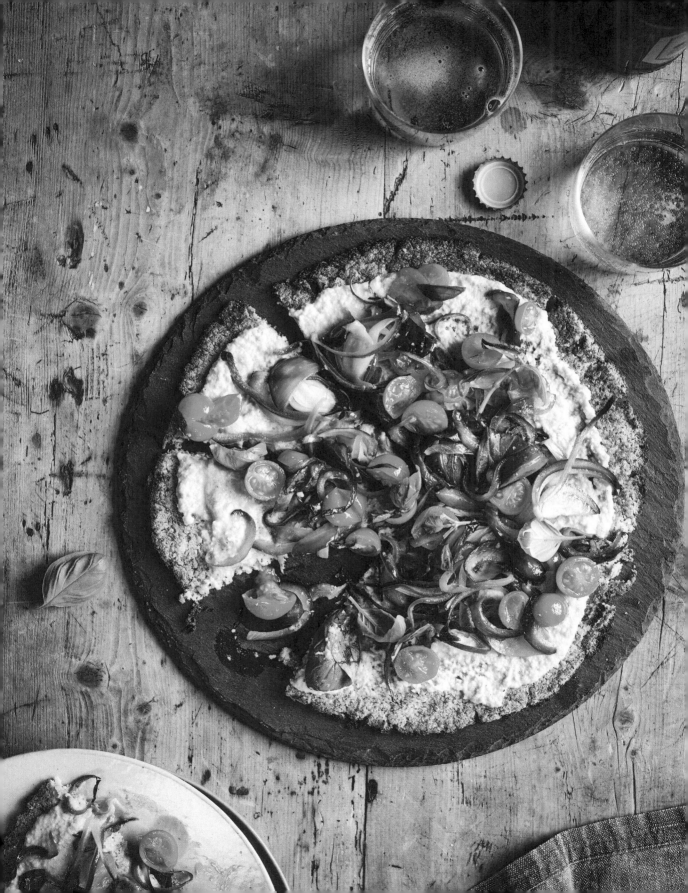

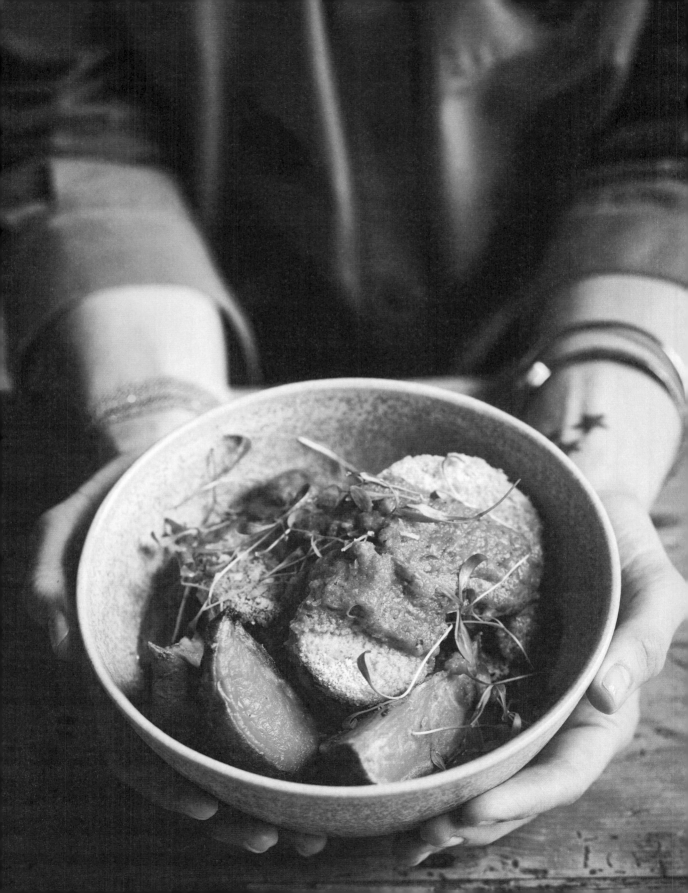

katsu curry

Katsu curry is one of my all-time favourite spicy numbers. Rather than just going for a chicken version I have also created an aubergine-based one (shown opposite) so you can pick and choose between the two. Instead of the usual coating of Japanese panko breadcrumbs, which contain wheat and can be irritating to the gut, this recipe is a grain-free version using a crust of almonds and coconut.

Super easy and super hearty, this goes really well with some sweet potato wedges or perhaps some of my Celeriac and Courgette Crispy Fries (page 177). Fluffy quinoa is another smashing accompaniment, or a green leafy salad if you want a lighter option.

serves 2

50g coconut flour

1 organic free range egg, beaten

50g ground almonds

4 tablespoons desiccated coconut

Generous pinch mineral-rich salt

2 organic free range chicken breasts, approx. 200g each

or

1 aubergine, sliced into 1.5cm-thick rounds

katsu sauce

2 carrots, peeled and roughly chopped

1 tablespoon onion powder

½ teaspoon garlic powder

1 teaspoon ground turmeric

2 teaspoons garam masala

2 tablespoons dried curry leaves

2 tablespoons coconut aminos

3 tablespoons unsweetened coconut yogurt

200ml organic Chicken Bone Broth (see page 57)

¼ teaspoon mineral-rich salt

Generous pinch black pepper

Preheat the oven to 200°C/Gas 6. Line a baking tray with baking parchment.

You will need three wide shallow bowls to create three dipping stations: put the coconut flour in the first bowl, the beaten egg in the second, and in the third combine the ground almonds, desiccated coconut and salt. Going through each of the stations in that order, dip either the chicken breast or the aubergine slices in each bowl and place on the lined baking tray. Bake in the oven for 25–30 minutes until crispy.

While these are cooking, make the katsu sauce. Steam the carrots for 10 minutes until tender. Add the cooked carrots to a blender with the rest of the sauce ingredients and blend on the highest setting. Transfer into a saucepan ready for warming.

Remove the chicken or aubergine from the oven. Leave the chicken to rest for 10 minutes and then cut into slices across the wider part of the breast. Warm the katsu sauce for 3 minutes, stirring constantly, and pour a generous serving over the chicken or aubergine.

tip

If the aubergine is large, you may need to increase the quantities of the crust ingredients.

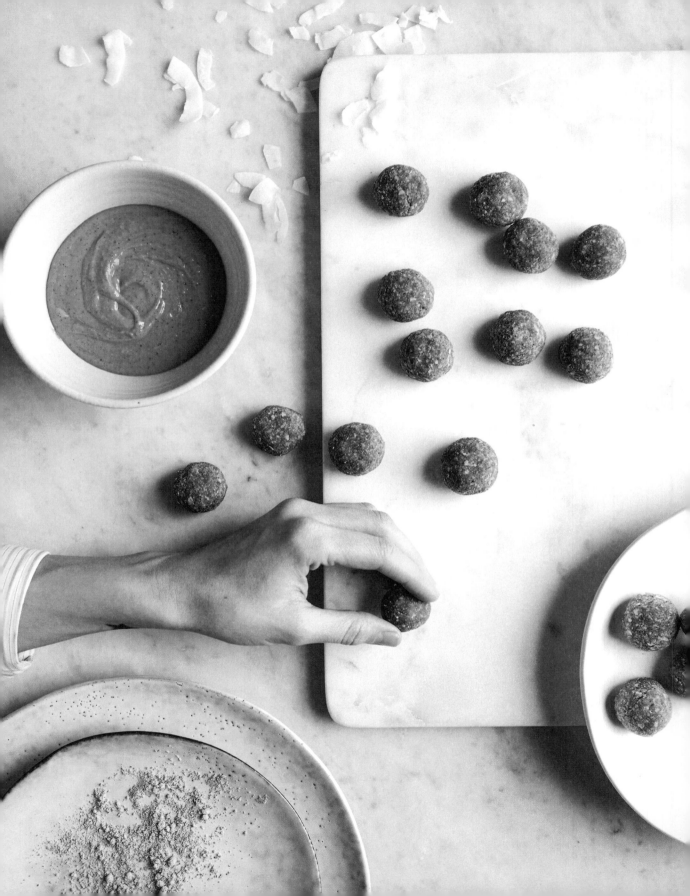

7

the gut saboteurs

JUST AS EVE couldn't resist the forbidden fruit in the Garden of Eden, we can so easily be swayed into eating foods that we know we really shouldn't. Food has never been so readily available and temptation is all around us. Whether it's a quick fix on the way home from work, a home-delivered pizza for the third night in a week, a daily sugary treat – because your afternoon cuppa just isn't the same without it – or too many glasses of wine in the evening, we often succumb to our own inner serpent.

So why is it so easy to fall off the wagon when we try to break bad habits, even when we have the best of intentions? What drives our patterns of behaviour and causes us to revert to old habits? According to psychologists, it takes between one and three months to change

a habit and most of us don't give ourselves enough time or space for that. In addition, there are very real psychological and emotional reasons why we gravitate towards certain things: succumbing to temptation isn't simply a question of being 'weak willed'. Physical factors also drive cravings, so it may be that it is your gut, more specifically your microbiome, that is convincing you to reach for that extra slice of cake or pizza when you know you shouldn't.

In this chapter we'll look at the role of the microbiome in our propensity to eat 'junk' foods. We'll also examine the part that other factors, such as stress, certain medications and a lack of sleep, can play in sabotaging the gut and our microbiome. You'll be pleased to see, however, that you can still enjoy naturally sweet foods that will give your taste buds a hit but without the sugar crash. My delectable collection of ice creams (see page 183) demonstrate that and will be a revelation. And if you're a lover of those ubiquitous sugary cereals, my Hazelnut, Cardamom and Cacoa Granola recipe on page 174 will ensure you are never tempted by the sugary, shop-bought stuff again. Burgers are also well and truly on the menu with my delicious Happy Cow Burgers (page 180).

sweet seduction

Alright, so we know sugar isn't good for us. The campaign mounted by the 'sugar police' over the last couple of years has made sure of that. But, joking aside, there is no denying that more and more research has linked high consumption of sugar with detrimental effects to our health. We know this, so why do we continue to be enthralled by its sweetly seductive taste?

The answer partly lies in our biology. We have a primal instinct to eat foods that are high in sugar. In Palaeolithic times they provided our ancestors with a valuable source of instant fuel – handy if you needed to quickly refuel to chase a boar, but not quite so good today, when we have sugar at our fingertips 24/7. The crucial point is that these types of food – and remember in those days sugary food meant seasonal fruit, not cookies and muesli bars – were once few and far between so human beings didn't develop a biochemical mechanism to tell us when to stop eating them. We simply don't know when enough is enough.

You don't have to go back very far to see the massive transition in the types – and amount – of sugar we eat. Just two generations ago, something as simple as fruit was eaten as a special treat. Contrast that with the high amount of concentrated juice and abundance of sugary snacks we now eat on a regular basis.

Our addiction to sugar can also be blamed, in part, on the craze for low-fat diets that began a couple of decades back. We were encouraged to ditch fat because it was blamed for increasing our waistlines. So, dutifully, we bought low-fat foods, thinking they were the healthier option when, unbeknown to us, we were simply trading fat for a shed load of sugar. Saturated fats were deemed to be the chief villains in this campaign, despite the fact that they are necessary for things like the production of hormones, supporting metabolism and gut health, as well as keeping us satiated. What is apparent now is that, ironically, this demonisation of fat made us hungrier and fatter than ever. It's really not the case that fat makes you fat. Excess sugar does this, since we are designed to metabolise only a certain amount of sugar before the body stores the rest in fat tissue.

When people talk about the detrimental effects of sugar they're usually referring to fructose, one of its components. A spoonful of table sugar is made up of 50 per cent glucose and 50 per cent fructose. Glucose can be used for immediate, readily available energy and is, in fact, the prime source of fuel for the body's cells. This is metabolised rapidly, mostly by the gut. Fructose, in contrast, bypasses the gut and goes straight to the liver, where, rather than being used immediately for energy, it is converted into fat. For our Palaeolithic ancestors this would have been a good thing, and particularly beneficial for when we wanted to store up energy for a rainy day, but fast forward to our current lifestyles and it just means we are piling on unnecessary pounds.

sugar is sugar is sugar

OK so we know we should limit the amount of cake, biscuits and sugary treats we eat but unfortunately sugar isn't always easy to spot or indeed avoid. It can crop up in the most unlikely places – in sauces like ketchup and soups and even in foods such as bread or prepared salads. Labelling is hard to decipher as well. Even when the label says 'no added sugar', it might be lurking in a different guise. Often we can be hoodwinked into thinking we are making a better choice by opting for 'healthy' options such as granolas, fruit juices and muesli bars when really they are just sugar bombs in a different form.

Sugar can also appear in forms that many mistakenly believe are much healthier than the white stuff. Let's look at some of these in more detail.

Syrups You might have been misled into thinking some of these are healthier than the white stuff, but they have much the same effect. That's why I like to call them 'the pretenders'. Dollop a whole load onto a so-called 'healthy' granola and you have a sugar frenzy just waiting to happen.

There are loads of these products on the market: familiar ones like golden syrup, treacle and maple syrup, as well as the more unusual varieties like coconut or agave. But let's not kid ourselves, in essence they are all the same. It doesn't matter if they are 'naturally derived' from tree sap, like maple, or cacti, in the case of agave, they all equate to the same thing – too much fructose. Some have a lower GI status, which means that they don't raise your blood sugar levels quite so quickly and create such a wham-bam effect, but they still all contain fructose.

Note that I haven't included honey in this group. While the processed 'fake' junk from the supermarkets is exactly like the syrups above, as we saw in Chapter 4 (page 96), raw unrefined honey does have nutritional benefits and, when consumed in moderation, helps support the immune system and gut.

Artificial sweeteners What's not to like about something that's sweet, provides zero calories and was once heralded as the perfect solution for weight loss? Yes, I'm talking about those colourful little packets you might have seen people using in their coffee or tea. As it turns out, artificial sweeteners, including aspartame, sucralose and saccharin, have some pretty grim side effects that include messing with your metabolism and nervous system. Plus, they spell disaster for our gut microbes, altering their composition in an unfavourable way.

Stevia has recently become the 'en vogue' sweetener, so you might be thinking it's the perfect option. Think again! Although it is technically derived from a plant, and it doesn't raise blood sugar levels or contain fructose, it can often be just as processed as artificial sugar substitutes. If you are going to use it, ensure it is taken from whole leaf or raw extracts.

Xylitol is a sugar alcohol that you see in a lot of health food products and sugar-free gum. This is derived from birch bark but by the time it has been manufactured one has to question how 'natural' it really is. Natural or not, xylitol can create digestive issues so perhaps the gut is telling us something there.

why sugar is bad for the gut

So what of our microbiome in all this? How is it affected by a high intake of sugar? Well, given that microbes enjoy a feast of fibre, which sugar and sweeteners (with the exception of fruit) do not provide, sugar doesn't really do it for our microbes. However, microorganisms such as *candida albicans* love the stuff, as well as other types of bacteria (we'll look at these more in Chapter 9). Excessive consumption of sugar can feed the growth of these more disruptive microbes and when unchecked this can lead to an overgrowth that compromises the flourishing of beneficial microorganisms. When yeasts like *candida albicans* are able to take hold they can also damage the gut, as they attach themselves to the intestinal barrier and may contribute to leaky gut.

These sugar-loving microbes are clever in their quest to get their 'fix' in that they can increase cravings for sweet foods, so it becomes a self-perpetuating cycle and makes the need for sugar all the more insatiable. It makes sense for them to do this, to increase their chances of survival, but it is not good for our bid to quit sugar or restore balance in the gut. That's why cutting out sugar isn't always a straightforward process. We also need to simultaneously nourish and bolster our microbiome in order to get this back in check, and that includes sugar cravings. Often these can indicate a microbial imbalance rather than just a weakness for raiding the biscuit tin. The Weed, Seed and Feed programme on page 46 can help you to support your microbiome, as well as guide you on how to avoid refined sugars and manage cravings with naturally sweet alternatives.

what about fruit?

This is where I have a major problem with the anti-sugar movement, as fruit has been caught in the crossfire in the obsession with cracking the habit. It has been shown that fruit, in moderation, does not to have the same effect as highly concentrated sources of sugar since its fructose content is nowhere near as high. More to the point, when you eat fruit you also take in fibre, which slows down the absorption of sugar, as well as a wealth of vitamins and minerals. However, even with fruit, moderation is important. We don't need more than one or two pieces of fruit per day so, with your morning smoothie for example, don't be tempted to load up on fruit and pop in a token bit of spinach at the end. Too much fruit ultimately equals too much fructose.

how to get sugar addiction under control

The first step is not to include too many sweeteners as a regular part of your diet, so as well as going easy on the white stuff, be mindful of those mentioned in the box on page 167. You also need to be a bit more aware of all those misleading 'healthy' foods such as granolas, fruit juices and muesli bars. It is actually better to have a piece of cake that is freshly made, with whole ingredients, once in a while than to regulary eat those 'healthy' snack bars that are high in sugar – natural or otherwise. You might want to cut out sugar entirely for a short period. If so, follow my Weed, Seed and Feed programme. However, the long-term strategy should be to thoroughly and whole-heartedly enjoy that slice of cake as a treat but not eat lots of sugar on a regular basis.

In order to achieve that you may have to retrain your taste buds and your microbiome not to crave sugar in the first place, and that means finding other ways to give added flavour to your food. Spices such as cinnamon and vanilla will

it's all in the label ... or is it?

We know that our microbes don't like sugar but they would also turn their noses up at the thousands – yes thousands – of artificial and unpronounceable ingredients that are lurking in our food. Labels are an altogether confusing matter, which is ironic given they are supposed to provide clarity. Terms like 'natural', 'original' and 'traditional' might sound reassuring but technically they don't mean anything, so while you might think you are buying into something wholesome, that's not always the case.

However, there are other much more sinister ingredients that we need to watch out for, including preservatives such as sodium benzoate and artificial trans fats such as partially hydrogenated oils. The latter are liquid fats to which hydrogen gas has been added to make the oil solid at room temperature (to turn it into a margarine, for example), thereby changing the entire chemical structure. These artificial trans fats have been linked to many health conditions, including heart disease and diabetes. And of course let's not forget all the artificial preservatives and flavours in processed foods – these can have similar health implications when consumed regularly. Because of mass food manufacturing these kinds of chemicals have made their way into the modern diet in a big way and cumulatively they can have consequences.

So how do you avoid them? Start by buying foods in their most natural state, not boxed, bagged and complete with cooking instructions. Another good rule of thumb is if you don't recognise an ingredient as a food, or if your grandmother wouldn't know it as food, then put it back on the shelf. There are too many chemical shape shifters in processed foods, which put an added burden on the gut and its microbial army, so try to prepare your own meals from scratch where possible.

provide a flavour kick, and coconut milk and its flesh add a natural sweetness without the side effects of regular sugar. Give my coconut milk-based ice creams on pages 183–185 a go.

This isn't about never having sugar again, but adopting a more mindful approach as to why and how you are using it. Understand your cravings and manage those, rather than looking for a sugar replacement. Your cravings might be driven by microbial imbalances in the gut or triggered by an emotional need (more likely a combination of the two), so find ways to 'reward' yourself that don't involve a sweet pick-me-up. Create 'feel good' rituals, such as enjoying a really nice herbal tea (liquorice

is great as it is naturally sweet) or finding something to fill your time when you know that a craving will kick in – going for a walk, doing a yoga class or simply having a relaxing bath.

Understanding and embracing the times when you have the urge to go crazy on the stuff is an important part of changing your habits. If you try to eliminate sugar for ever you will just make yourself entirely miserable – and it's unnecessary. It's about having much more of a holistic approach and changing your mindset for the long term. And never forget that your microbes have much more to do with those cravings than you ever thought, so supporting your gut should be a fundamental part of controlling that inner sugar fiend. It might be incredibly tempting to sail down the chocolate river into the land of candy but as Violet Beauregarde, who turned into a giant blueberry in *Charlie and the Chocolate Factory*, would tell you, it isn't really worth it in the end.

medication nation

Let me make one thing clear before I look at some of the drawbacks of certain medications: modern medicine is life-transforming and, of course, life-saving, and it has achieved incredible things in recent decades. But the reality is that excessive medication can create some serious turmoil for our microbiome and our gut.

Much of the problem lies with unnecessary medication. Reaching for ibuprofen at the slightest hint of a headache or chucking back antacids when we could have simply chewed our food more thoroughly are common quick fixes that easily become a habit. Most people have no idea that certain types of medication – including NSAIDs (non-steroidal anti-inflammatory drugs), such as ibuprofen, and other meds like antacids – can have negative effects. These include stripping the body of essential vitamins, minerals, antioxidants and beneficial bacteria, all of which can lead to more symptomatic side effects and more medication. Crucially, these drugs can also compromise the barrier of the gut, increasing the likelihood of leaky gut and creating more inflammation over time. Next time you are about to go for the 'sticking plaster' approach and pop a pill, remember that doing this too often can soon catch up with you, and unfortunately your gut and microbiome suffer the brunt of it.

That said, the real grenades to the microbiome are antibiotics. They are incredible at fighting life-threatening infections but there's no doubt that until very recently they have been given out like Smarties. Aside from the issue of growing levels of antibiotic resistance, taking countless antibiotics has the catastrophic effect of destroying many of our beneficial microbes. This leaves the gut susceptible to an overgrowth of pathogenic microorganisms and yeasts that have the potential to create ongoing issues for the gut and our general health. So the important thing is to use these medications only when you really need them.

Our obsession with 'cleanliness' isn't limited to medication. In our overly sanitised society we are consistently compromising our health with anti-bacterial soaps, household products and sprays. Microbes outnumber us remember, and, as the famous microbiologist Louis Pasteur once said, 'It is the microbes that will have the last word.' Bear that in mind the next time you reach mindlessly into the medicine cabinet or are tempted to wipe down your entire home using an anti-bacterial cleaner.

is your mind working overtime?

Gut saboteurs don't just come in the form of food and other substances we put into our bodies. As we saw in Chapter 5, the brain–gut connection is a powerful one and sometimes the mind is the biggest hurdle in our journey towards gut health.

take a little time

The chances are you are reading this with your phone within glancing distance, mid-way through answering an email while

For too many of us, eating has become more of a chore than a pleasure ... we rush back to scrolling through endless social media or furiously texting on our phones.

simultaneously knocking back a cup of coffee. We are officially addicted to distraction. In a world where we have never been so connected on many levels, it's all too easy to become disconnected and fail to make meaningful connections with each other or the food we eat.

For too many of us, eating has become more of a chore than a pleasure and rather than spend time preparing and enjoying a meal we rush back to scrolling through endless social media messages or furiously texting on our phones.

Our default setting tends to be a state of 'fight or flight' but in that flurry of excitement, grabbing food on the go and bolting it back with little thought, we can never optimise our digestion and switch into the 'rest and digest' mode that can be so beneficial to the gut. If we are not present with the food on our plate and fail to allow the processes of digestion to work properly then we cannot expect our gut to function at its best. Moreover, with a bit of planning and preparation we undoubtedly make better choices with our food, rather than mindlessly opting for the same old sandwich from the same chain every day.

My clients often say that they don't have time to eat healthily, and with busy lifestyles that include numerous work and family commitments, admittedly time is precious. But we all have time. You simply need to alter the way you use it. Is spending hours on social media, for example, so important? Prioritising and a bit of planning will free up time. Taking the time to think about your

shopping list means you don't end up over-filling your supermarket trolley and then throwing away perfectly good food at the end of the week. This also saves pennies. Dedicate an hour each Sunday to making a meal plan for the week ahead and prepare some things in advance that you can have to hand when you come in from work late or need something healthy and quick in the morning. Try baking my Super Seed Bread (page 157), Broccoli and Walnut Bread (page 226) or Cinnamon Loaf (page 224). They are all super-tasty, easy and I would go as far as to say cathartic on many levels – the aroma of them baking in the kitchen is enough to make you feel pretty smug about having dedicated a bit of time to your food. Other great time-saving ideas include boiling eggs for the week ahead or whipping up soups with double portions for freezing.

Once you are in the right place to start making changes I suggest you embark on a bit of a kitchen pantry detox since physically clearing space makes for a clearer mind too. Having those sneaky cream crackers lurking at the back of the cupboard can make even the most steely minded among us succumb to temptation, so get rid of them. If they're not there you can't eat them. Once you've done a spring clean, fill your cupboards and fridge with wholesome, flavoursome and downright awesome foods. (See my shopping guide, on pages 260–267, which will help you get started.)

Giving your mind a clearout is an important part of this. It's time for a digital detox. That doesn't mean being totally evangelical and switching your phone off for days on end, although some report that as the most liberating thing they have done in years, but more having boundaries on when you are 'online'. A 9pm curfew on digital devices is a good rule of thumb as it allows your natural circadian rhythms to kick in, which promotes better sleep. Most of us struggle to get a good night's sleep and this has its own implications for the gut. Here's why …

i can't get no sleep

The lyric above, from one of the most well-known 90s club classics, is a sentiment that many people will sympathise with. Insomnia is incredibly common, with a soaring number of us sleeping for a mere 5 hours per night, when we should be aiming for closer to 8 hours. Most of the reasons for tossing and turning in the night are down to worrying and stressful life events. We then compound that by stressing about being less effective the following day. However, the effects are much more serious than that. Missing out on decent shut-eye leaves us exhausted but it also has a major impact on our health and gut.

Studies show that the circadian rhythms that govern our sleep–wake cycles are very much in tune with the daily rhythms of gut bacteria. As we saw in Chapter 5, there is a powerful brain–gut link and many of the positive neurotransmitters, like serotonin, are produced by the microbiome. Crucially these chemicals don't simply support your mood but also govern your sleep. In fact, melatonin, the main hormone needed for healthy sleep, is created in the gut as well as the brain and can operate on its own rhythm, independent of its pineal counterpart. Moreover, deficiencies

in intestinal melatonin have also been linked to increased intestinal permeability or leaky gut, which as we discussed in Chapter 4, has its own effect on the gut. In the same way that microbes play a significant role in managing our sleep, they can also be disrupted by a lack of shut-eye. Studies have shown that people with jet lag or poor sleep patterns experience a shift in their microbial rhythms which results in metabolic disruption, glucose intolerance and weight gain. It's a two-way relationship: our microbiome needs the rest and rejuvenation and likewise it helps support better slumber.

Creating a pre-bedtime ritual will help if you suffer from insomnia. Switch off your phone (the blue light it emits promotes brain activity) and give the emailing, surfing and texting a rest for at least an hour before hitting the sack. And definitely never do any of these things in the bedroom. There are only two things you should be doing there and shopping online isn't one of them. Instead, use that hour to have a bath, read, write a journal or meditate, anything that helps you wind down.

And while working late at night cannot always be avoided, you can take control of your mealtimes. Don't save up your 'rations' until the end of the day and have a mighty feast when you get home. That will mean you need to stay up really late with your digestion working overtime or, if you go to bed within a couple of hours of eating your feast, you'll end up with a whole lot of food sitting in your gut overnight. Soups like my Spicy Parsnip Satay Soup (page 83) or Carrot and Coconut Chermoula Soup (page 203) are a great go-to if you know you'll need to put in the extra hours at your desk in

wine

Ah, wine – the proverbial 'elephant in the room' as far as nutrition is concerned. There often comes a point in consultations when the client apprehensively asks me, 'So, are you going to tell me not to drink wine?' The answer to that is almost always a resounding 'No, of course you can drink wine – in moderation.'

But before you swiftly pour yourself a glass of vino, here are a few interesting things to consider. Until fairly recently, wine was made without chemical intervention, whereas synthetic sulphites and other substances are now often added to most commercial wines. Sulphites are generally used as mild antioxidant preservatives and stabilisers. They occur naturally in many foods, but not at the levels you will find in a bottle of plonk. To put it in perspective, one egg contains 6 ppm (parts per million) whereas a standard glass of wine has around 350 ppm, most of which are chemical derivatives. The process of fermentation does produce sulphur dioxide but it is man-made sulphites that cause the strong reactions in some people. So some of the blame for a heinous hangover could lie with the high amount of sulphites in your favourite choice of vino.

Biodynamic and 'natural' wines use minimal technological processing and are free from synthetic chemicals and additives. Typically these tend to be organic, sustainable and produced by small-scale vineyards. They can be hard to spot as many of the makers cannot afford to put their products forward for official certification, and, technically, there is no universal definition when it comes to 'natural' wines. However, if you do a bit of research, you will be able to get hold of them (see page 261), and many restaurants that champion seasonality and sustainability will have them on the menu. Here's the best bit though, our microbes also seem to like a bit of a tipple, too. Maybe it's the polyphenols in the wine (red or white) or it could be the bacteria produced during the fermentation process. Or perhaps, just like us, they might need to take the edge off a bit given all the miraculous work they do.

the evening. Huge salads are not ideal. Too much raw food at night can be more taxing on the gut so aim to have that earlier in the day.

be kind to yourself

There are many potential saboteurs and it can be difficult to avoid them completely, but discovering the factors that can knock you and your gut off course has, I hope, made you feel a whole lot more empowered. Recognising and knowing how to manage those saboteurs is what really counts, and doing the best you can, as often as you can. No one is perfect and it's very important to give yourself a break from time to time. Be kind to yourself. If you strive for perfection and are overly self-critical you can be your own worst saboteur. You have the power to change patterns of behaviour and now the knowledge and the recipes to get you started.

hazelnut, cardamom and cacao granola

The aroma of this delicious granola wafting through your kitchen will have you wanting to dive head first into this sweet and spicy flavour combo. Using activated nuts and seeds (as explained on page 16) is not only more digestion friendly but makes this even more nutritious as your body can access all of the bountiful vitamins, minerals and proteins available. I use raw honey as a binder, which gives a great depth of flavour and I believe is one of the better sweetener options. Serve this with your milk of choice, either raw or organic unhomogenised dairy milk or a plant-based milk – my fave is Hazelnut Milk (page 151). Kefir also works well. Allow it to soak into the granola and eat with delight for a gut-friendly start to the morning.

makes about 350g (approx. 7–8 servings)

130g activated hazelnuts
45g activated pecans
65g activated cashews
30g activated pumpkin seeds
30g activated sunflower seeds
20g coconut chips
25g cacao nibs
2½ tablespoons raw honey
1 tablespoon melted coconut oil
1 teaspoon ground cinnamon
1 teaspoon ground cardamom
1 teaspoon fennel seeds
Seeds from 1 vanilla pod
3 generous pinches mineral-rich salt

Preheat the oven to 150°C/Gas 2. Line a baking tray with baking parchment.

Place the activated hazelnuts, pecans, cashews, pumpkin seeds, sunflower seeds, coconut chips and cacao nibs in a food processor. Pulse for 30 seconds to break down a bit into smaller chunks, but not too fine. Transfer to a large bowl.

Add the honey, coconut oil, cinnamon, cardamom, fennel seeds, vanilla and salt. Mix thoroughly until well coated. Transfer to the baking tray and bake for 20 minutes, then give it a bit of a stir and pop back in for a further 15 minutes. Alternatively, you can use a dehydrator at 46°C for 24 hours.

Store in a sealed glass jar in a cool dry place or the fridge.

tip

Add a generous dollop of coconut yogurt with a drizzle of raw honey if you want an extra indulgent brekkie.

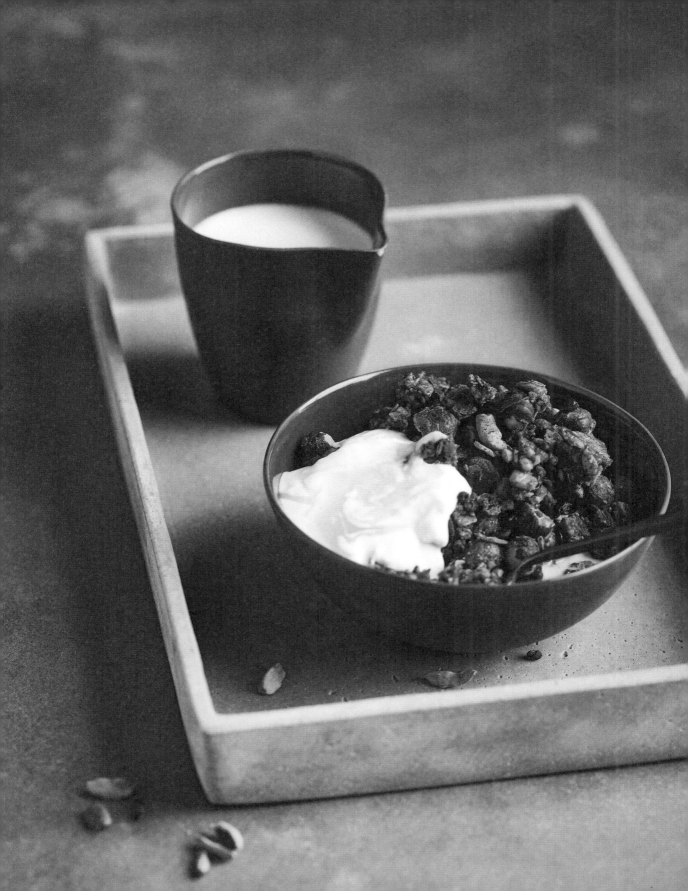

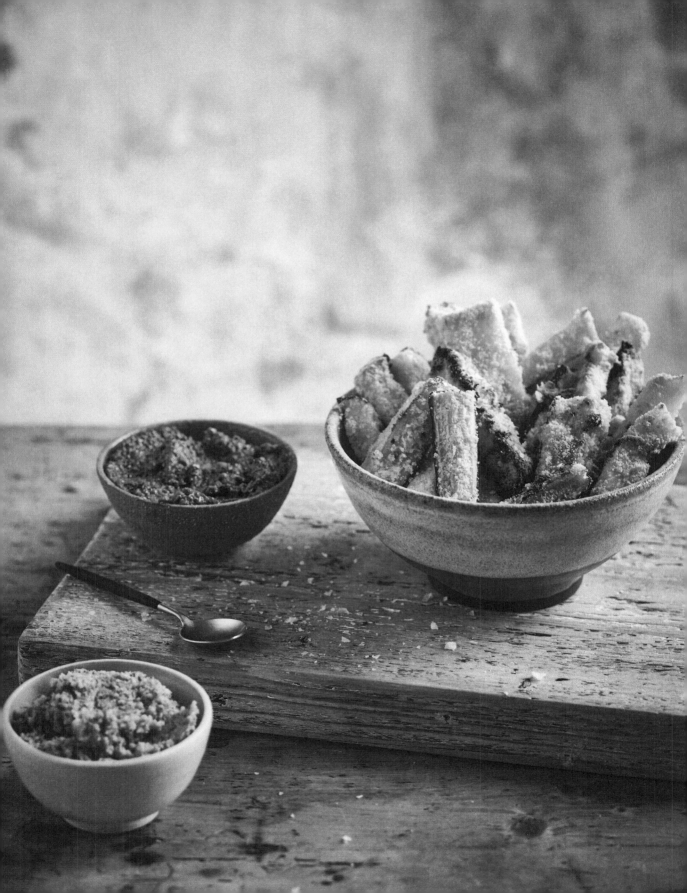

celeriac and courgette crispy fries

These are a take on regular fries with an almond crumb to give them a distinctive crunch and avoid the deep frying and nasty trans fats that you will find in many potato chips – one of the major gut saboteurs in so many ways. Try dunking them in my Broccoli, Almond and Artichoke Dip (page 29) or Raw Beets Dip (below).

serves 3–4 as a side

1 celeriac trimmed, peeled and cut into 7.5 x 2.5cm batons

2 courgettes, trimmed and cut into similar size batons

50g ground almonds

¼ teaspoon mineral-rich salt

Preheat the oven to 200°C/Gas 6. Line a baking tray with baking parchment.

Place the celeriac and courgette batons in a steamer for 10 minutes. In a large bowl, combine the ground almonds and salt. Add the steamed veggies and coat thoroughly, then lay them on the baking tray and place in the oven for 30–35 minutes until crispy. Leave to cool for 5 minutes before serving.

raw beets dip

Beetroot has myriad benefits: it contains antioxidant compounds and is an excellent source of fibre for the gut. This recipe also uses raw garlic, one of the most potent prebiotic foods you can eat.

makes 1 small bowl

1 beetroot, peeled and roughly chopped

1 garlic clove, peeled

3 tablespoons fresh flat-leaf parsley

3 tablespoons tahini

3 tablespoons extra virgin olive oil

2 tablespoons unsweetened coconut yogurt

2 tablespoons pine nuts

1 teaspoon ground cumin

Juice of ½ lemon

½ teaspoon mineral-rich salt

Place all the ingredients in a food processor and blend until combined (it won't be entirely smooth). You may need to stop and scrape to get an even consistency.

Transfer to a sealable glass or ceramic container and store in the fridge for up to 3–4 days.

chipotle red pepper dip

Who doesn't like a spicy dip to add a colour pop to their plate? This one is truly flavoursome, with a deep smoky taste from the chipotle chilli and paprika. I created it as an alternative to ketchup, which can contain whopping amounts of refined sugar: I prefer to enjoy my sweet treats rather than find them creeping into condiments. As well as the red peppers, which are packed with antioxidants, this recipe uses tomato paste, one of the best sources of another antioxidant, lycopene, and together with tomatoes in their raw form they all help support the microbial activity and protective effect in the gut. This is a brilliant dip for Celeriac and Courgette Fries (page 177), but you have to try spreading it on top of Happy Cow Burgers (page 180) with a generous slice of unpasteurised halloumi. Delicious!

makes 1 small bowl

2 red peppers, halved and deseeded

3 tablespoons tomato paste

1 tablespoon extra virgin olive oil

3 tomatoes, roughly chopped

Pinch chipotle chilli flakes

2 teaspoons mild smoked paprika

1 teaspoon ground cumin

2 teaspoons onion powder

¼ teaspoon garlic powder

Generous pinch mineral-rich salt

Preheat the oven to 200°C/Gas 6. Roast the peppers in the oven for 20 minutes.

Leave to cool, then chop roughly and add to a food processor. Add all of the other ingredients and pulse to get a thick-textured dip.

Transfer to a sealable glass or ceramic container and store in the fridge for up to 3–4 days.

spicy nacho dressing

This Mexican-inspired creamy dressing is super-versatile and easy to make and it avoids a lot of the dubious ingredients you might find in a typical shop-bought dressing that are not so hot for our gut. Use it to pimp a plate of salad leaves or to dress some Nacho Kale Chips (see page 246). It also works really well drizzled over roast chicken, sliced avocado, sweetcorn and sweet potato for a Mexican bowl of goodness. This dressing is based on almond nut butter and uses nutritional yeast flakes to give it a cheesy flavour, so if you are vegan or just want to try a dairy-free dressing, then this is a winner!

makes 1 small bowl

2 teaspoons smoked paprika

1 teaspoon garlic powder or 1 garlic clove, peeled and crushed

2 teaspoons onion powder

2 teaspoons ground cumin

5 tablespoons (15g) nutritional yeast flakes

75g almond nut butter

Juice of 1 lemon

½ teaspoon mineral-rich salt

Place all the ingredients in a blender and blend on the highest setting, adding water if necessary to thin to a smooth, creamy consistency.

Transfer to a sealable glass or ceramic container and store in the fridge for up to 3–4 days.

tip

This is great with avocado on toast to give it a spicy Mexican kick.

happy cow burgers

I decided to call these Happy Cow Burgers because buying meat that is ethically, locally and organically produced is essential, as it contains higher levels of nutritients and the cows are treated with respect. In this recipe I have included mushroom extract, which not only enhances the umami flavour but also boosts the body's immune system. I love these burgers served with some baked sweet potato wedges or my Punchy Potato Salad (page 62). Another delicious and gut-friendly option is to use a large portobello mushroom as a bun instead of a white refined grain bun. I reckon choosing three tasty toppings makes a good burger into a great burger and you can get super-creative with them. My favourite combo is thinly sliced unpasteurised gherkins, Sauerkraut (page 58) and a generous slice of unpasteurised Manchego. Avocado 'Mayo' (see page 87) or Chipotle Red Pepper Dip (page 178) are other tasty options.

makes 6 burgers

500g organic grass-fed beef mince

2 tablespoons tamari

3 tablespoons nutritional yeast flakes

2 generous pinches mineral-rich salt and black pepper

1 organic free range egg, beaten

2 teaspoons mushroom extract (optional)

1 handful fresh parsley, finely chopped

½ tablespoon organic unsalted butter or ghee

Place the mince in a large bowl with the tamari, yeast flakes, salt and pepper, egg and mushroom extract, if using. Add the parsley and mix together using clean hands. Try to handle as little as possible to avoid the meat becoming tough. Divide the mixture into six and shape into burger patties. Place in the fridge and leave to firm up for 30 minutes.

When ready to cook, preheat a large griddle or frying pan on a medium heat. Add the butter or ghee to coat, then cook the burgers for 4–5 minutes on each side. Serve hot, with your choice of toppings and sides.

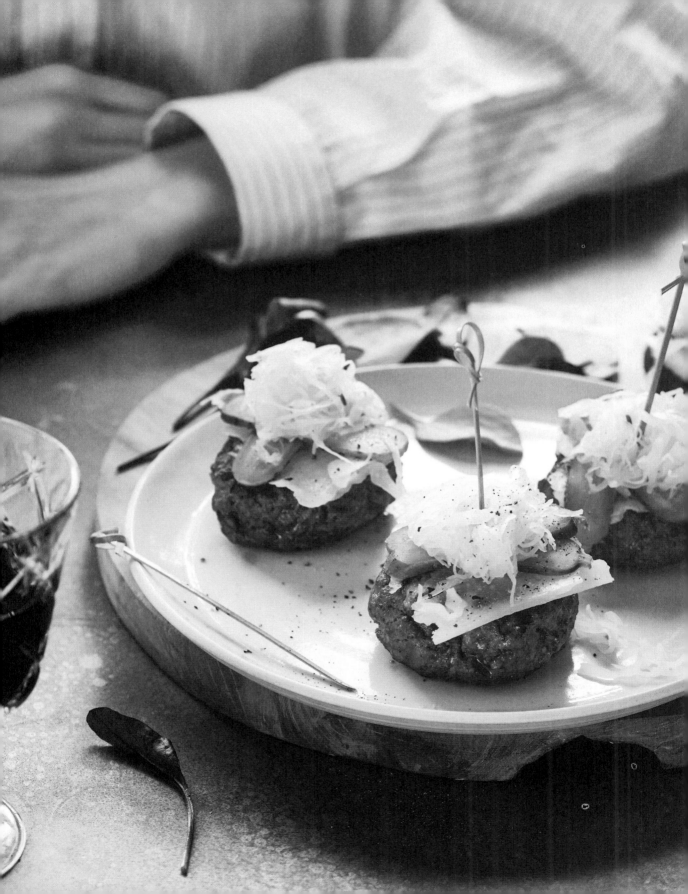

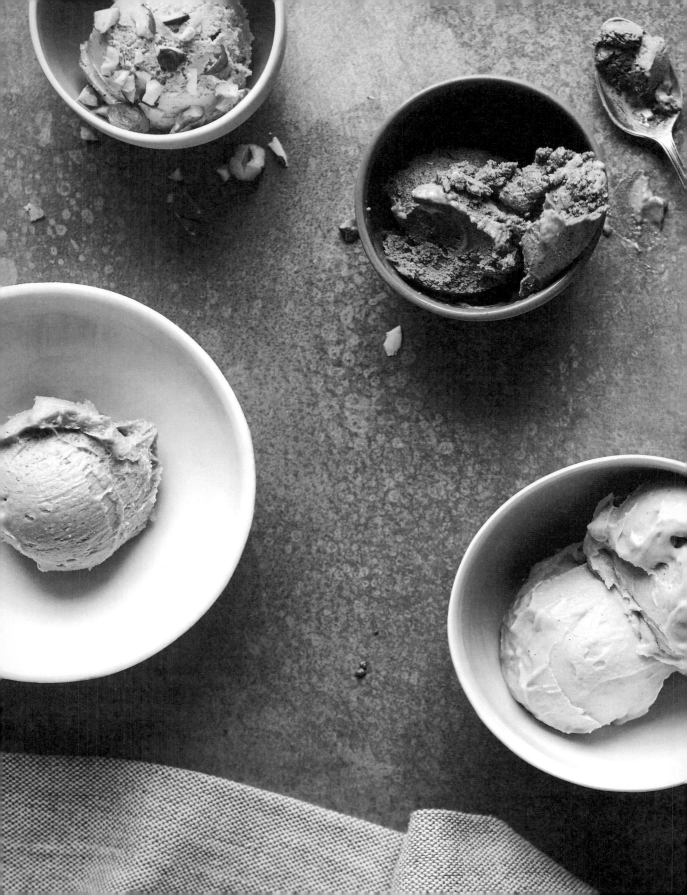

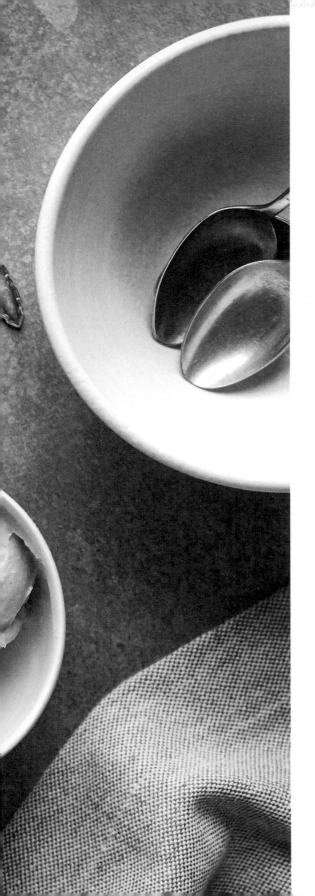

the ice creams

I LOVE ice cream. But it's all too easy to devour an entire pot and then have that sugar coma feeling afterwards. Not nice for you or your gut. With that in mind I set about creating a collection of ice creams that both your gut and your taste buds will love. They are based on full fat coconut milk and it is important to understand that certain types of saturated fat, such as coconut, are incredibly soothing for the gut. What's more, they are naturally sweet, which means you don't need to add any sugar. I've picked some of my favourite flavours for the following four recipes and genuinely find that a modest scoop is totally satisfying and hits the spot. But it is also fun to serve them knickerbocker glory style for a real treat.

amandino ice cream

160g cashews, soaked for 2 hours
45g flaked almonds
2 tablespoons white almond nut butter
200ml full fat coconut milk
Seeds from 1 vanilla pod
Pinch mineral-rich salt

Drain the cashews and thoroughly rinse with filtered water. Place in a high-speed blender with all of the other ingredients and blend until smooth. You will need to use the tamper to push down the ingredients and/or stop and scrape to get this evenly smooth.

Pour into a glass or ceramic container and freeze. Your ice cream will be frozen in 1 hour.

Take it out of the freezer 20–30 minutes before you want to eat it, to allow it to soften.

nocciola ice cream

190g cashews, soaked for 2 hours
3½ tablespoons hazelnut butter
200ml full fat coconut milk
Seeds from 1 vanilla pod
Pinch mineral-rich salt

Drain the cashews and thoroughly rinse with filtered water. Place in a high-speed blender with all of the other ingredients and blend until smooth. You will need to use the tamper to push down the ingredients and/or stop and scrape to get this evenly smooth.

Pour into a glass or ceramic container and freeze. Your ice cream will be frozen in 1 hour.

Take it out of the freezer 20–30 minutes before you want to eat it, to allow it to soften.

bitter choc ice cream

makes approx. 400g

190g cashews, soaked for 2 hours
3 tablespoons cacao powder
3 tablespoons cacao nibs
1 teaspoon shavings of white cacao butter
200ml full fat coconut milk
Seeds from 1 vanilla pod
Pinch mineral-rich salt

Drain the cashews and thoroughly rinse with filtered water. Place in a high-speed blender with all of the other ingredients and blend until smooth. You will need to use the tamper to push down the ingredients and/or stop and scrape to get this evenly smooth.

Pour into a glass or ceramic container and freeze. Your ice cream will be frozen in 1 hour.

Take it out of the freezer 20–30 minutes before you want to eat it, to allow it to soften.

rose and cardamom ice cream

makes approx. 400g

250g cashews, soaked for 2 hours
4 teaspoons rose water
2 teaspoons ground cardamom
1 teaspoon beetroot powder
200ml full fat coconut milk
Seeds from 1 vanilla pod
Pinch mineral-rich salt

Drain the cashews and thoroughly rinse with filtered water. Place in a high-speed blender with all of the other ingredients and blend until smooth. You will need to use the tamper to push down the ingredients and/or stop and scrape to get this evenly smooth.

Pour into a glass or ceramic container and freeze. Your ice cream will be frozen in 1 hour.

Take it out of the freezer 20–30 minutes before you want to eat it, to allow it to soften.

kombucha matcha float

Kombucha is a sweet and fizzy fermented green tea; once you try it you will be hooked. Like other fermented foods, kombucha is made from a starter culture of bacteria. In this case a SCOBY (symbiotic culture of bacteria and yeast) transforms into this delicious drink. It's great on its own and a good substitute for a glass of wine at the end of a long day but I also love it in this rather impressive-looking dessert for entertaining friends on a summer's evening. You can also eat the matcha ice cream on its own. I use white cacao butter in this recipe (obtained from cocoa beans that are pressed to remove the cocoa solids) as it's a healthy source of saturated fat and gives a decadent flavour to the ice cream. Check out page 262 for info on where you can buy this.

serves 2

200ml full fat coconut milk
190g cashews, soaked for 2 hours
Seeds from 1 vanilla pod
1 tablespoon matcha
1 teaspoon shavings of white cacao butter
40g desiccated coconut
Pinch mineral-rich salt
400ml kombucha

Put all the ingredients, except the kombucha, into a high-speed blender and blend until thick and smooth. You will need to use the tamper to push down the ingredients and/or stop and scrape between blitzing. Transfer to a glass or ceramic container and put into the freezer for at least 1 hour to set fully.

When you want to make the floats, take the frozen mixture out of the freezer and leave for 30 minutes to soften slightly.

Divide the kombucha between two glasses and then using an ice-cream scoop add a generous scoop of the matcha ice cream to each glass. Enjoy with a spoon and straw.

chai bites

These are great for when you need a pick-me-up as the warming chai spices are immediately soothing. While these are treats, they use dates as a sweetener so the gut also has a fix in the form of fibre. These bites go perfectly with a loose-leaf black tea infused with cardamom pods.

makes approx. 20 bites

125g activated cashews (page 16)
25g flaked almonds
40g desiccated coconut
½ teaspoon mineral-rich salt
Pinch black pepper
Seeds from 1 vanilla pod or ½ teaspoon vanilla powder
1 teaspoon ground cinnamon
2 teaspoons ground turmeric
¼ teaspoon ground cardamom
¼ teaspoon ground ginger
120–140g pitted dates

Place all the ingredients, except the dates, in a food processor and pulse until you have a fine dough-like texture. Then gradually add the dates until the mixture binds well. Add a tiny amount of water if you need to.

Remove from the machine and roll to about 1cm thick, then cut into bites. Store in an airtight container in the fridge for up to 4 days.

orange blossom sake-tini

Your eyes do not deceive you … this is indeed a cocktail recipe. As you will probably have gathered, I believe that a healthy approach to food and drink means everything in moderation. As with food, it is really a question of being a bit more discerning about the types of alcohol you consume. Premium sake, for example, can act as a good digestive tonic in small amounts. I've paired it with fragrant orange blossom water and the rich sweetness of pomegranate molasses for a fresh and uplifting mix. Here's to good health and a tipple once in a while!

serves 1

100ml premium sake
½ teaspoon pomegranate molasses
1 teaspoon orange blossom water
Orange peel shavings

Add ice to a cocktail shaker then add the sake, molasses and blossom water and shake. Pour into a martini glass and garnish with the orange peel shavings.

gin booch fizz

A fragrant and fizzy combo of kombucha (a fermented green tea) and delicate gin, made even more delicious by the addition of fresh herbs. It's simple to make and even better to drink.

serves 1

1 measure gin
100ml kombucha (see page 186)
1 tablespoon fresh lemon juice
Couple of sprigs of rosemary
and thyme

Pour the gin into a glass, add the kombucha and lemon juice and lightly stir to mix together. Add the fresh herbs and a couple of cubes of ice.

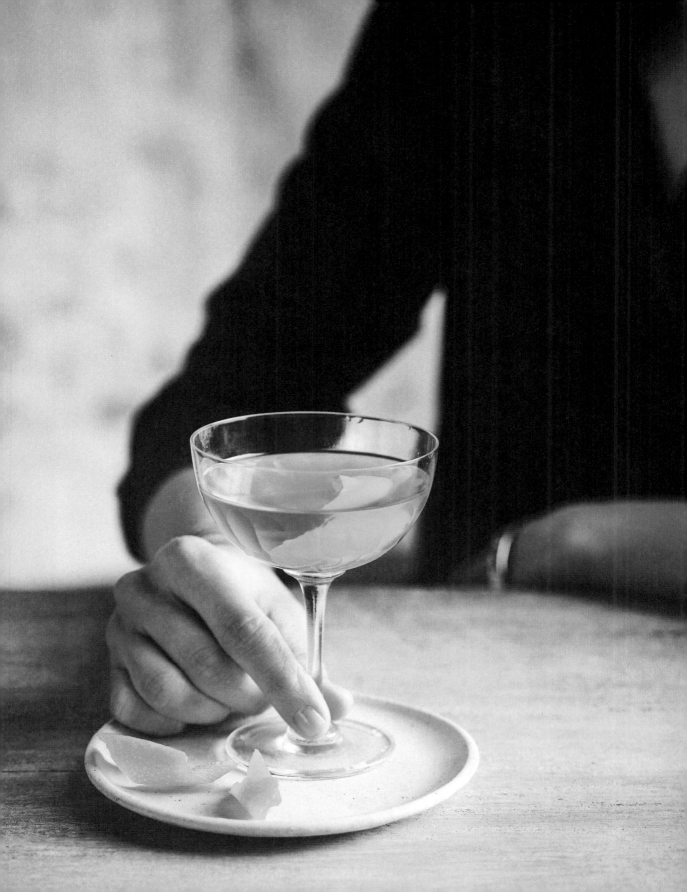

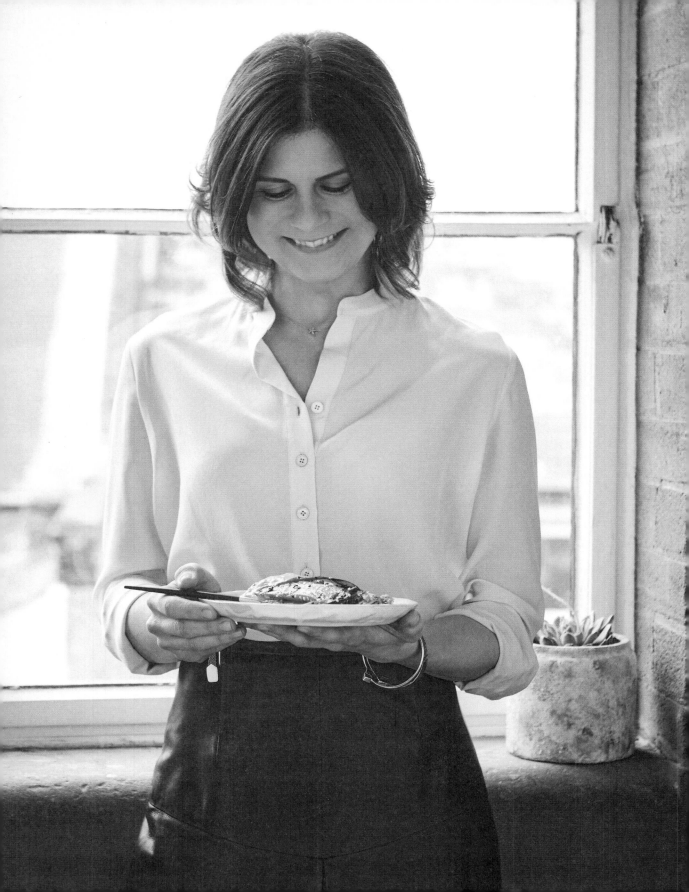

CHAPTER 8

wired and tired

PICTURE A HAMSTER on a wheel, never quite knowing when it might be able to get off, just relentlessly running, running ... and running. This sums up how many of us often feel. Living in a crazy, challenging and chaotic world means that we are constantly on our toes, jumping from one thing to the next with little respite, to the extent that our bodies just can't keep up. In fact, the consequences of chronic stress have been linked to just about every modern disease you can think of – from depression through to autoimmune diseases and numerous digestive conditions.

Only in the past few decades has life become so unbelievably intense. We are under constant pressure to have successful careers, be perfect parents, exercise regularly, eat well, make time for friends, look our best and, on top of all that, appear totally calm and collected. And being plugged in to our phones and other devices means we are never offline. It is unsustainable and we know it.

All that plate-spinning leaves no down time, which means zero space for the body to recharge and recoup. Chuck in the side effects of poor sleep, one too many skipped meals, sugary snacks and endless cups of coffee and you are well on your way to being a major stress head.

As we saw in Chapter 5, the brain and the gut have an intertwined relationship so it should come as no surprise that the gut is one of the first places to feel the effects of a fast and furious lifestyle. This chapter is all about the impact stress has on the gut. I'll look at what the fight or flight response means from a physical perspective, the role of our adrenal 'stress' glands and the knock-on effects of all this on the gut and the microbiome. I'll also provide practical advice on managing your stress through making lifestyle changes and choosing foods that can help bring you and your gut to a more calm state. Recipes like my Karma Krackers on page 210 (it's all in the name, folks), Pink Porridge on page 200, and one of my absolute faves, Shiitake, Leek and Seaweed Broth (page 204), pack in a whole heap of naturally relaxing foods. So with a cup of soothing Turmeric Chai Latte (page 211) in hand, let's begin.

the fight or flight response

Before we look at stress in detail it's important to understand that it isn't always a bad thing. In acute situations, stress is a primal instinct that helps us to meet and overcome challenges in our environment.

'Fight or flight' is a mechanism by which the brain tells the rest of the body that it needs to switch up into 'stress' mode to respond to a threat. Physically this starts with a perceived stressor that activates the HPA (hypothalamus–pituitary–adrenal) axis. The hypothalamus and pituitary gland are both located in the brain; the adrenal glands sit just above the kidneys. Once the HPA axis is activated it sends a message to the adrenal glands to flood the body with stress hormones that include cortisol and adrenaline, preparing the rest of the body either to fight for survival or flee the perceived danger. Blood rushes to the muscles, digestive processes are halted, heart rate is increased and glucose is

mobilised for energy. In essence we are all set for a battle or to run.

This can be a life-saving mechanism during a crisis, but it is meant for short, sharp bursts and not the chronic activation that happens multiple times per day for many people. Moments like someone aggressively barging past you to get on the bus, sitting in a traffic jam when you're already late or receiving a hideous email from your boss are just a few examples of situations that can get you worked up into a mini frenzy.

The fight or flight response is automatic, regardless of whether the stressor is positive or negative. Even something positive like exercise can put the body into a momentary state of stress. However, when this stress response reaches a chronic state, it can become overwhelmingly negative.

Our working days are longer than ever – some might say never-ending, due to modern technology. This puritanical work ethic means we are pushing ourselves way beyond our limits to the point where it is catching up with us on a physical level. The problem with constantly treading water in this way is that other bodily systems, such as the immune, reproductive and digestive systems, become almost 'secondary' and therefore are not always able to do their jobs properly. You are hardly going to stop for a spot of lunch if you are running for your life: the body sees digestion as somewhat arbitrary in its quest for survival and this is why the gut is so susceptible to the effects of chronic stress.

stress will make you sick

As we saw in Chapter 5, the brain–gut connection operates on a feedback mechanism, constantly relaying all sorts of information back and forth. Stress is a big part of this and stressors will also directly affect the functioning of the gut. Just as the brain tells other parts of the body to mobilise for an attack, it also gives our gut a warning so our internal army is prepared for the onslaught. This information is passed from the brain, via the vagus nerve, to the microbiome and the enteric nervous system in the gut, which is why you might get a nervous, nauseous feeling there when you are stressed. This stress response, and the release of associated hormones, can alter the bacterial composition of the gut and as such compromise our microbiome. This negative shift can also impair the growth and diversity of our beneficial microorganisms, which may have a far-reaching impact on our immune system and the level of inflammation in the body.

It may also compromise the intestinal barrier and promote leaky gut, which can compound an already stressful situation. Chronic stress almost always leads to an inflamed, irritated and stressed-out gut.

To make a bad situation worse, stress hormones like cortisol affect insulin (the blood sugar hormone) levels. When stress hormones are chronically activated, it can lead to a bit of a metabolic mess that promotes insulin resistance, which impairs how efficiently the body shuttles glucose into our cells to be used for energy. Therefore we will crave high-sugar foods to raise our depleted energy levels. This is why we feel drawn to these foods when we are under chronic stress. However, that sugar fix leads to further disruption in the microbiome, starting a whole cascade of negative effects in the gut. It therefore becomes a stress- and sugar-induced vicious cycle.

Conversely, skipping meals will also have a knock-on effect with cortisol as the body thinks it is starving so triggers a stress response that further raises blood sugar levels. Therefore regular balanced meals with adequate protein is fundamental to keep this in check, as protein helps to slow down the release of glucose from carbohydrates, thereby making energy release more consistent. Furthermore, stress can alter the production of hydrochloric acid in the stomach, making it higher or lower, and that also compromises the way we are able to digest our food. This often means that reflux symptoms can be more pronounced during stressful times. Additionally, stress has been associated with a reduced production of all gastric secretions, which impairs the way in which we absorb nutrients from our food, and compromises the functioning of the gut.

We have to understand that when it comes to stress there is a gut–brain feedback loop, so a simultaneous strategy of supporting the gut *and* reducing factors that are causing stress is the only long-term solution. Our stress glands, the adrenals, play an important part in this feedback system, so let's take a closer look at these walnut-size powerhouses that work so hard to keep everything under control, and the consequences of pushing them too far.

adrenal overdrive

You may have heard about the phenomenon of 'adrenal fatigue'. The more accurate term for this is HPA axis dysfunction and it reflects an imbalance of cortisol production. (This is very different from Addison's disease, a life-threatening state of adrenal insufficiency, or Cushing's syndrome, in which the body produces excessive amounts of cortisol.)

As explained earlier, the HPA axis is activated when we come into contact with a perceived stressor. The adrenal glands then release the stress hormones that prepare the body to respond physically by fighting or fleeing. This process is part of a normal stress response, but when the HPA 'switch' is consistently flicked, our adrenals start to tire. Typically this will lead to chronically elevated levels of cortisol, adrenaline and other stress hormones, as the adrenals frantically pump away in response to a persistent state of alarm. This results in that stereotypical 'adrenaline junkie' feeling.

However, what goes up must come down. The adrenals eventually go into a downward spiral, as they simply can't maintain the production of hormones at the required level. This represents the 'fatigue' part of the term 'adrenal fatigue'. When the adrenals reach this low point, symptoms such as poor sleep, decreased libido, low mood, sugar or salt cravings and persistent tiredness are common. There is also often a propensity for weight gain, particularly around the middle (sometimes referred to as 'the cortisol tyre').

In addition, the thyroid and the reproductive organs may suffer as they both interact with the HPA axis; thyroid conditions and fertility issues may be linked to adrenals that are struggling to cope. (See Chapter 9 for more about these issues.) And of course the gut also becomes chronically 'tired', because imbalances in our stress hormones have negative implications for our microbes, as mentioned above.

But all is not lost. The crucial thing is to recognise that you are burning the candle at both ends *before* you reach the point of exhaustion, by which time it is harder to correct the imbalances in your hormones and gut. So if

you are pretty wired most of the time, you need to take action.

Saliva tests (see page 269) can give you an indication of how your cortisol levels are looking, but we all know intuitively whether we have pushed the boundaries too far. We simply have to learn to acknowledge our limits, although that can be hard in a society that is perpetually 'driven'.

adrenal stressors

Much like a credit card, you can't keep maxing out on your adrenals. You also need to have a savings account that is regularly topped up, and this means minimising some of your outgoings. There are a few things that will really pummel the adrenals. Let's examine the major culprits.

Coffee Glugging back endless cups of coffee might seem like a good idea when you start to feel a drop in energy and it may temporarily keep you revved up throughout the day. However, caffeine is a stimulant that directly affects the adrenals and sooner or later overexposure to these high-octane hormones will have a negative impact. That would be crash and burn! For most people, one or two cups a day is usually OK. Since your stress hormones should naturally be at their highest in the morning, you don't want to raise them further with a double shot of espresso as soon as you hit the alarm button. Having your coffee after breakfast or mid-morning, when you have a bit of food in your belly, is a better option as the caffeine then doesn't have the same jump-start effect on the adrenals.

Alcohol At the other end of the day you might be so wired when you finish work that your natural inclination is to pour a large glass of wine to help you relax. Now wine, in

salt

Some research has linked consumption of salt to a host of health problems, including high blood pressure and degenerative bone conditions. While it's true that excessive intake of the salt found in processed and junk foods, as well liberally adding generic table salt to your food, isn't good for us, this is the type of salt that has been stripped of its nutrients, leaving only sodium chloride. It certainly isn't the more naturally derived stuff that comes from the sea or earth, which has an abundance of minerals and trace elements; this unadulterated salt provides us with crucial minerals that work together to support fundamental processes in the body. The heart, muscles, nervous system and absorption of food depend on these minerals. In short, the human body wouldn't be able to function without salt. Alongside sodium and chloride, these natural salts contain other minerals such as magnesium and calcium and perhaps as many as 85 trace elements in some varieties.

Salt has always been an important part of our diet, but in a world of processed foods we are consuming a lot more of the 'empty' kind. Ironically this has left our diet depleted in nutrients that would naturally be present if we were seasoning real food in its most natural state with pure, mineral-rich salt.

You don't have to buy into the hype of getting pink salt from the Himalayas. In fact, opting for a salt that is found close to your geographical area is not only healthy but often less expensive and more environmentally friendly. Of course we can overdo it, even with the nutritious versions, but a pinch of mineral-rich salt can enhance the flavours on your plate *and* give you a health boost.

moderation, has its nutritional benefits, but if you have spent too much on that adrenal credit card by drinking it regularly to calm your system, you may need to curb your consumption for a while. Alcohol isn't kind to the adrenals. That isn't to say you can't enjoy the odd glass now and then, but giving due consideration to your adrenals when you know they are at tipping point will serve you well in the long run.

Poor sleep Another biggie for depleting the adrenals is poor sleep. Sleep is your opportunity to recharge your batteries and if you don't replenish the tank with enough fuel then you can't go very far. Good quality sleep is therefore essential for managing stress and has an impact on how our gut microbial rhythms work, too.

Most of us are familiar with those nights spent tossing and turning, ruminating about a project deadline or family issue, so it is important to make your nightly pre-bed routine a priority. Have a look at page 172 for tips on how to maximise your pillow time.

Sugar Of course you are going to want to reach for a sugary treat if you're feeling stressed, but don't fool yourself. Sugar in any form gives the adrenals a bashing, due to the knock-on effect it has on cortisol and insulin, as mentioned above, as well as on the gut, so try to avoid these quick fixes. The initial sugar high is invariably followed by a resounding plummet.

During periods of stress you may also crave salty foods. This may be due to disruption in the body's sodium balance as the adrenals play a role in managing this. As with many other foods, there are some serious misconceptions about the effects of salt on our health. We *do* need it, but we also need to be mindful of where we get it from and how much we eat (see page 195).

rest and digest

The journey to a less wired and tired system begins with the foods that we eat and the way that we consume them. Shovelling down your dinner while standing by the fridge checking your email isn't a relaxing way of eating, irrespective of how nutritious the food is. See Chapter 1 on how to eat more mindfully.

Having said that, there are a number of foods that can help support a stressed-out system, including mineral-rich salt and naturally salty foods. Rather than diving head-first into a packet of Pringles, though, try including more of the natural sources of salt such as miso, seaweeds, artichokes and of course a pinch of the good stuff (see page 195).

You also need to support natural anti-inflammatory processes to restore your body to a calmer state. One of the best ways to do this is by increasing your intake of omega 3 oils, which are found in oily fish such as wild salmon, mackerel and sardines, organic grass-fed or pasture-raised meat and poultry, and flaxseed, chia and hemp seeds. Omega 3 oils are essential fatty acids – 'essential' means they cannot be produced by the body so must be ingested – that help to reduce inflammation, resulting in a less overburdened system.

Healthy fats in general will help us maintain a more composed frame of mind since they actively nourish our neurons (brain cells),

supporting smoother communication channels in the grey matter, rather than the frantic 'firing off' that happens when we are in a state of nervous panic. The brain is made up of a high percentage of fat and gut microbes appreciate healthy fats too, since these support their anti-inflammatory role. Think coconut milk, coconut oil, ghee or organic butter and avocados. Cold pressed oils, such as extra virgin olive oil, are great too, but use them in dressings rather than for cooking, as high temperatures alter their chemical structure, meaning that they can generate free radicals rather than provide health benefits.

We also know that our gut microbes love fibre. In fact, when it comes to stress, fibre is nectar for the microbiome. Eating plenty of fibre from a wide variety of foods allows the bacteria in the colon to produce compounds such as butyrate, a short-chain fatty acid that has a pivotal role in reducing inflammation. The soluble fibre found in many vegetables is the dish of choice for these bacteria. It's found in foods such as sweet potatoes, cooked and fully cooled white potatoes, sourdough, sprouted oats, unripe bananas, apples and ground flaxseed, to name a few (for more on this, see Chapter 2). Whatever your choice, you need a daily intake of fibre to support a less stressed gut.

Vitamin C is another a key nutrient for reducing stress as it is used up readily to produce cortisol and other stress response hormones. Some of the best food sources are peppers, broccoli, chillies, green vegetables strawberries and kiwi fruit.

Last but not least, magnesium is top of the league when it comes to calming the nerves – and it is a mineral that our body tends to use up in vast quantities during stressful periods. You'll find it

avocado

They say 'cool as a cucumber' but when it comes to calming foods, the avocado wins hands down. This deliciously creamy fruit has a gazillion hashtags on Instagram and a cult following for a reason.

Firstly, it contains decent amounts of important minerals such as relaxing magnesium and potassium, which helps the body to manage sodium levels (which are often disrupted when the adrenals are struggling to keep up). Its natural anti-stress make-up also includes several B vitamins, particularly B_5, one of the major vitamins for adrenal health, and it boasts good levels of vitamin C and healthy oils – both fundamental to managing stress. This powerhouse food also contains anti-inflammatory compounds and it is rich in antioxidants, those protective phytochemicals that prevent cell damage. And, on top of all that, avocados are a great source of soluble fibre, which our microbes love. So get your guacamole at the ready; avocados just hit the anti-stress jackpot!

As well as adding avocado to salads and sandwiches, try my avo-inspired recipes such as Raw Tacos (page 207), or for a sweet treat my Avocado 'Nutella' Cream (page 115), and let's see if you don't feel a lot more chilled.

herbal tonics

As well as adapting your diet to help alleviate the effects of stress, you could consider introducing a herbal tonic. Let's take a quick look at a bunch of plants that have been renowned for many centuries for their energy- and immunity-boosting properties. These are known as adaptogens, and helping us adapt to stress in our environment is exactly what they are famous for doing.

These herbs are believed to have a protective and restorative function in the body that includes negating the negative effects of high levels of stress hormones, increasing the natural buffers your body uses to combat stress-related damage and promoting sleep. They appear to be able to 'turn up' or 'turn down' the body's response depending on where your internal stress 'thermostat' is hovering. How brilliant is that?

So what are these magical stress busters? One of the best known is liquorice root, which can be steeped in teas or taken in tincture form. Other adaptogens include the roots of rhodiola, astragalus and ginseng. In Ayurveda, traditional Indian medicine, ashwagandha root and holy basil are often used for their anti-stress, fatigue-fighting and immune-boosting properties. We can also include medicinal mushrooms here, particularly cordyceps, which perform a similar stress-management role. (You can read more about the amazing benefits of mushrooms on page 100.)

When it comes to taking adaptogens, the ideal formula is one that combines a few of them, because they all have slightly different roles. However, it is important to consult a registered nutritional practitioner or your doctor before you go ahead with supplementing.

in nuts and seeds, leafy greens, sprouted grains and avocados. In fact the mighty avocado deserves a shout out as an antidote to stress (see page 198).

Above all else, and before you dose yourself up on herbs and avocados like they are going out of fashion, it is vital to realise that nothing, and that really means *nothing*, will protect you from chronic stress unless you adapt your lifestyle. For many people, this can be the hardest part of making a positive change, as slowing down can feel totally counterintuitive. Think about how wounded animals find a place to be still and allow themselves to heal. We humans need to do the same, but we seem to have lost the capacity to rest, and indeed digest.

slow the pace

There are a variety of ways of managing stress but mindfulness is one of the most effective in encouraging our natural healing process. Currently a buzzword in popular culture, mindfulness is still seen by some as 'mumbo jumbo' but you would be wise to embrace it.

But what does mindfulness actually mean and how does it have a role in gut health? Mindfulness is about being more present in your life generally, being mindful of what you are doing at the moment you are doing it and not being engaged in three things at once. Taking time to look around and breathe in your surroundings, rather than tapping away on your phone, can be a basic way of practising mindfulness. And its effect on the gut? Well, as mentioned in Chapter 1, the way that you eat has a marked impact on how you digest, and being present with what's on your plate is an important part of this, so master the art of how to eat using the guide on pages 19–25 to help your gut find that restful place during each and every meal.

Being consciously aware of the situations and the people in your life and understanding how they impact on your sense of wellbeing are also vital. This is where we really need to tune in to that inherent 'gut feeling' and identify and ditch the energy vampires! You know who and what these are in your life. They are the people and patterns of behaviour that suck the *joie de vivre* from you. I'm talking about those who stress you out, the takers that never give back and the repetitive self-sabotaging types of behaviour that you know in the end make you feel rubbish. It is time to be true and honest with yourself – and others – about what really matters to you and gives you pleasure and fulfilment. Get rid of the doubters and disbelievers and enrich your life with people who really listen who appreciate you warts and all. Learn to say 'no' to the things you know don't serve you well and instead leave you drained. The self-empowerment of connecting with what truly makes you happy and having the guts (excuse the pun!) to know when to walk away from a situation or not agree to it in the first place will also help to keep your mind, body, soul and of course your gut in harmony.

Lists, however, do not encourage harmony. Abandon the 'to do' lists and avoid the temptation to create endless tasks that you are unlikely ever to complete. Instead use that time to focus on what you are doing in the moment. 'Mono-tasking' is usually a lot more rewarding than multi-tasking. When we have multiple things on the go we rarely feel satisfied with any of what we set out to accomplish.

Be focused and fearless in your pursuit of happiness. Creating vision boards can be a good way to do this. Portraying your thoughts, ambitions and dreams through the means of illustrations, photos, anything that represents where you want to go and what you want to achieve, will help you to see the bigger picture of what you want your life to look like. If nothing else, the time spent doing something fun and creative will be relaxing.

And in all this healthy escapism, try to find a place where you can connect more spiritually on a daily basis. That doesn't mean that you have to go all voodoo about it or start chanting away on a cushion. Rather, find something that allows your mind to be free of mundane 'stuff' and create that essential headspace. It might be yoga, Pilates or meditation, all of which are proven to be effective in managing stress and improving digestive health. Even simple activities like washing up can leave your mind open to just letting thoughts and feelings pass in and out without overthinking and analysing everything. In his book *How to Eat*, Thich Nhat Hanh talks about how washing dishes can become a meditative experience if it is done with mindfulness. He also says, 'Chew your food, not your worries', which is pretty genius if you ask me, and a good reminder not to take things too seriously. There is a famous saying that 'laughter is the best medicine' and I'm sure there is also something in the phrase 'belly laugh' that means the gut likes a good chuckle.

be positive and appreciative

Positivity is more powerful than you realise. So give yourself a break, or a pat on the back when it's due, learn to give and receive equally and to have daily practices that transport you away from the humdrum and the pressures of life. That's not being indulgent in any way; it is an entirely necessary part of having a healthy gut for optimum wellbeing. Just find the techniques that work best for you.

The key thing to remember is that you need to tap into what feels right deep down in your gut physically and metaphysically. What is all that incessant drive for anyway? You need to appreciate what you have right here, right now, that's true, real and honest. And that starts from what's on your plate through to how you give back to yourself emotionally. So turn the speed dial down a few notches and go a bit slower.

There is an international Slow Food movement that is dedicated to the concept of taking time, care and effort in the preparation of dishes. Recipes like my Harissa Lamb-Stuffed Cabbage Rolls with Feta and Mint (page 253) can be wonderfully relaxing. Or try making my Beet and Fennel Burgers (page 208), which will not only nourish your gut with the anti-stress nutrients it needs but the prep time will allow you the space to connect with your food. The anticipation is worth it and you can perhaps bring that philosophy into your day-to-day life too, instead of being impatient for the next trend or fast fix. Remember the hare that wanted to run to the finish line, while the wiser tortoise followed the mantra of 'slow and steady wins the race' and became the champion. It's time to get off that wheel, stop and instead of running, do more living.

pink porridge

Pink foods immediately put a smile on my face and I'm sure many of you feel the same. The vibrant hue in this recipe comes from beetroot powder: it is just a powdered form of the vegetable. As well as a serious punch of colour, this powder gives a hint of sweetness and a boost on the nutritional front too. What's also really nice about this recipe is the sprouted buckwheat: it has a distinctive taste, rather like slightly burnt toast, and it provides a wealth of B vitamins and magnesium, both of which help to manage stress from a gut and a hormonal perspective. This is porridge with a difference that will start your day on a truly positive high note.

serves 2

80g sprouted buckwheat

3 tablespoons beetroot powder

6 activated Brazil nuts, roughly chopped (page 16)

40g desiccated coconut

1 teaspoon coconut oil

Generous pinch mineral-rich salt

200ml cashew milk (or use raw or unhomogenised full fat organic dairy milk, unsweetened almond milk or kefir)

100g unsweetened coconut yogurt, to serve

6–8 activated pistachio nuts, finely chopped (page 16), to serve

Put the buckwheat, beetroot powder, Brazil nuts, coconut, coconut oil and salt in a food processor and pulse for around 30 seconds to break up the nuts and buckwheat a bit. Then gradually add the milk to mix to a porridge consistency. You may need more or less milk to get your preferred texture, but don't add it all in one go or you may end up with a liquid mess.

In a small bowl, beat the coconut yogurt using a small whisk until you get a whipped consistency.

Divide the porridge between two bowls and serve with a dollop of the whipped coconut cream. Top with the chopped pistachios.

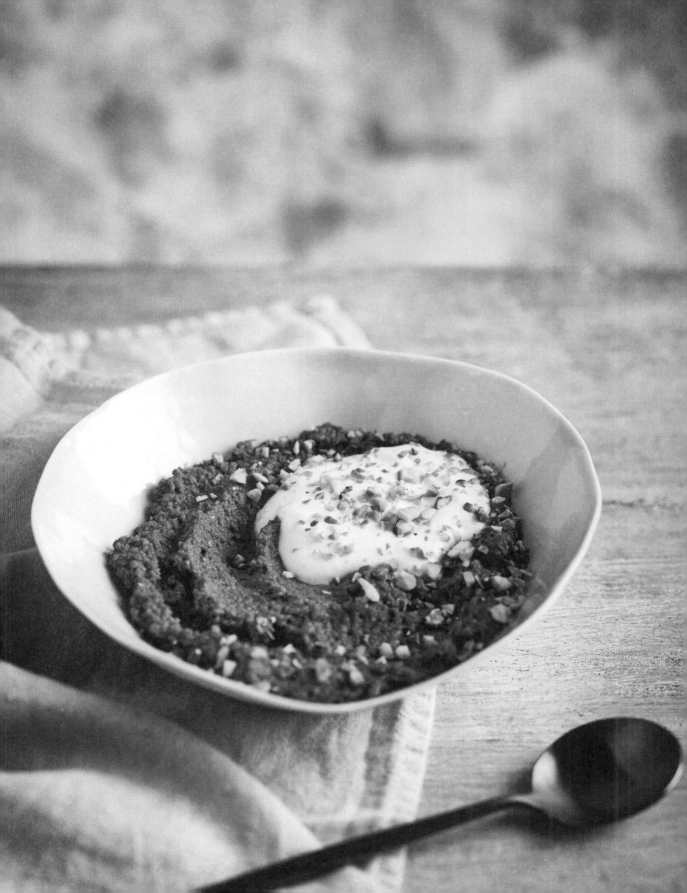

pear and hemp hearts smoothie bowl

Hemp hearts refers to the hemp seeds with their crunchy outer shell removed. This opens up these delicious seeds of goodness and all of the nutrition that they provide. Since they are a rich source of the essential fatty acids omega 3, 6 and 9 in an ideal ratio they help to provide crucial anti-inflammatory substances that keep the gut calm and collected. They are also a great source of fibre to help move digestive processes along smoothly. The flavour of these with pear makes a particularly tasty combo. A perfect stress-free start to the day.

serves 1

1 pear
¼ avocado
3 tablespoons shelled hemp seeds
8–10 activated cashews (page 16)
100ml milk of your choice: raw dairy milk, organic unhomogenised full fat milk, or unsweetened almond or cashew milk

Toppings
1–2 tablespoons crushed activated hazelnuts (page 16)
1–2 tablespoons coconut chips
1 tablespoon cacao nibs

Slice away a small section of the pear to garnish and put to one side. Then place the rest of the pear with all of the other ingredients in a high-speed blender and blend until thick and creamy.

Pour into a bowl and garnish with pear slices and a couple of the suggested toppings.

carrot and coconut chermoula soup

Chermoula is a spice blend that traditionally hails from North Africa; it combines beautiful sweet and smoky flavours that lift any simple soup recipe. Combined with carrots that are naturally soothing for the gut and turmeric that helps reduce inflammation, this soup will leave you feeling nourished and more balanced in mind, body and soul. Serve with a chunk of sourdough spread lovingly with ghee or organic unsalted butter. Feel-good food at its best!

serves 2

2 carrots, peeled and chopped

1 onion, peeled and chopped

1 garlic clove, peeled

2 tablespoons desiccated coconut

2 tablespoons tomato paste

2 teaspoons ground cumin

2 teaspoons ground coriander

½ teaspoon fresh ginger

1 teaspoon ground cinnamon

Pinch chilli powder

2 teaspoons smoked paprika

2 teaspoons finely chopped fresh turmeric (or ground turmeric, but the fresh stuff gives a more vibrant colour)

2 tablespoons chopped fresh parsley

Couple pinches black pepper

2 teaspoons mineral-rich salt

6 tablespoons (20g) nutritional yeast flakes

500ml organic Chicken Bone Broth (page 57)

Preheat the oven to 200°C/Gas 6. Line a baking tray with baking parchment. Place the carrots, onion and garlic on the baking tray and roast for 20 minutes.

While these are cooking, add all of the other ingredients to a high-speed blender. When the veggies are cooked, add them to the blender and pulse on high until smooth.

Pour into a saucepan and gently heat through, then divide between two bowls and serve.

shiitake, leek and seaweed broth

This is one of my favourite recipes, and it stands out for a few reasons. First, it incorporates so many gut-friendly foods – everything from prebiotic shiitake mushrooms through to fermented miso and organic chicken bone broth, with its healing amino acids. Shiitake mushrooms may also have a positive impact on managing our stress hormone levels to leave us less wired. The other key ingredient here is arame, a type of seaweed, which helps to support the growth of beneficial bacteria in the gut while crowding out the less friendly guys. Seaweeds are also high in protective antioxidant compounds as well as having a natural anti-inflammatory effect. This is a recipe that takes no time to prepare but gives you and your gut back tenfold. Serve with Karma Krackers (page 210) for a rejuvenating and relaxing steaming hot bowl of deliciousness.

serves 2

2 handfuls dried arame

1 tablespoon coconut oil

2 leeks, sliced

80g shiitake mushrooms, sliced

2 teaspoons finely chopped fresh ginger

6 thin slices fresh red chilli, finely chopped

1 garlic clove, peeled and crushed

3 tablespoons miso paste

4 tablespoons coconut aminos or tamari

500ml organic Chicken Bone Broth (page 57) (or use filtered water for a vegan version)

to serve

Sesame oil to drizzle

1 tablespoon Super Seed Mix (see page 127)

Handful fresh coriander, roughly chopped, or sprouts such as alfalfa, broccoli or radish

Soak the arame in cold water for 10–15 minutes, then drain.

Heat the coconut oil in a large saucepan and stir-fry the leeks for 2 minutes to soften slightly. Then add the mushrooms, ginger, chilli and garlic and stir-fry for a further minute.

Add the miso and coconut aminos or tamari and stir well. Then add the bone broth (or filtered water) and bring to the boil. Turn the heat down to low. Add the drained arame, loosely cover the pan and simmer for 10 minutes.

Divide the broth between two bowls. Drizzle with a little sesame oil, sprinkle with the Super Seed Mix and garnish with chopped coriander or sprouts.

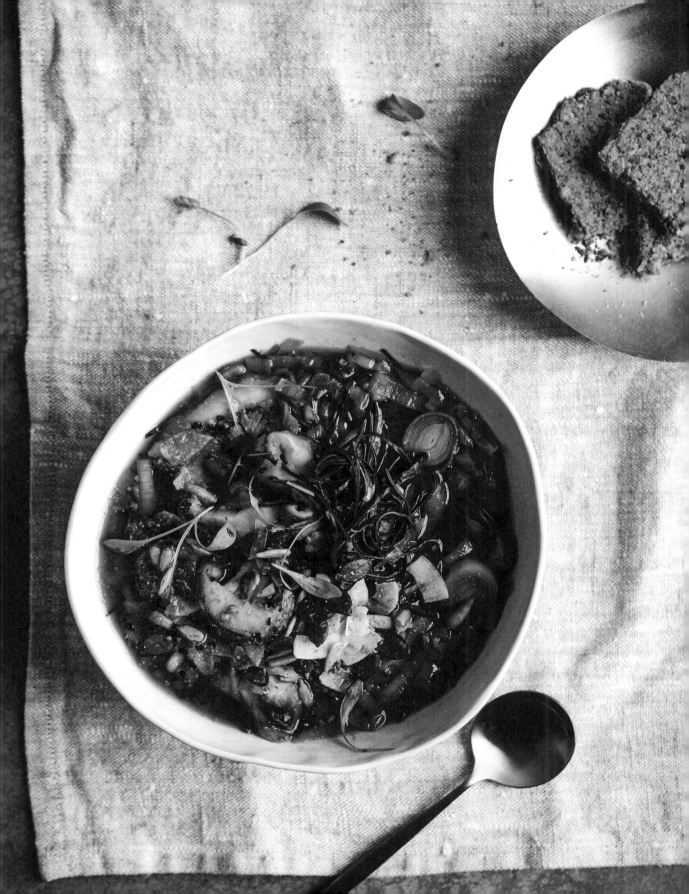

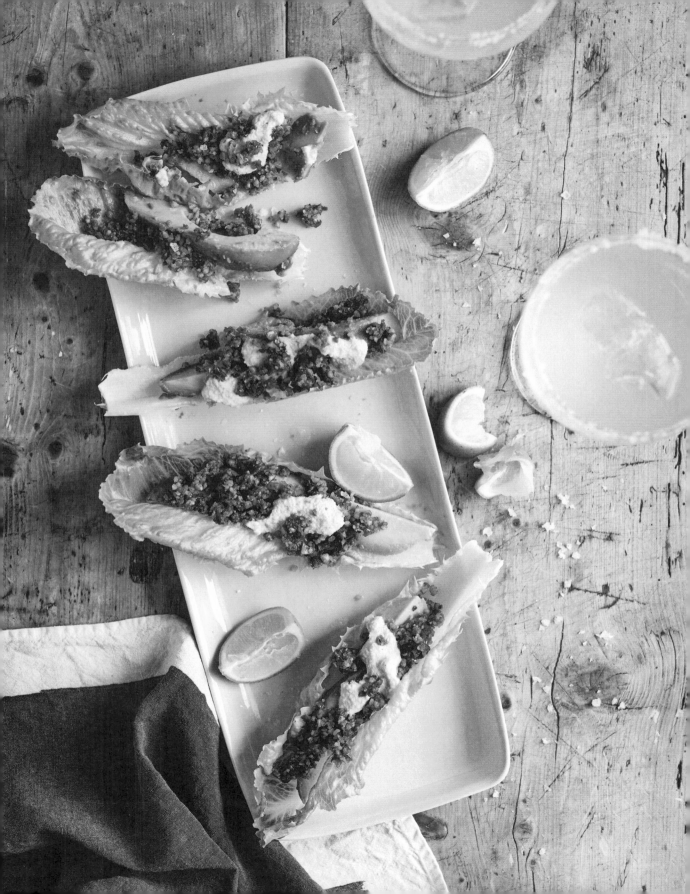

raw tacos

This taco recipe was inspired by a vegan friend of mine who is obsessed by Mexican food (including tequila cocktails) but wanted an alternative to beef tacos. Even though I'm not a vegan I have to say I think these are just as tasty as the meat version. To create the 'mince' I've used walnuts with sun-dried tomatoes and spices. Walnuts are one of the best sources of polyphenols – natural antioxidants that our gut microbes love – and it's always good to be mindful of your meat consumption in general. This is a great light lunch for summertime, and I often double or treble the quantities to entertain friends and family … and always with a pitcher of margarita on the side!

serves 2

8 small romaine lettuce leaves
1 avocado, cut into 8 slices
Fresh limes, cut into wedges

taco filling
50g walnuts
40g sun-dried tomatoes in oil (drained weight)
¼ teaspoon dried chilli flakes (I like chipotle best)
¼ teaspoon paprika
¼ teaspoon ground cumin
¼ teaspoon garlic powder
Pinch mineral-rich salt

cashew sour cream
30g cashews, soaked for 2 hours
Juice of ½ lemon
Pinch mineral-rich salt
50ml filtered water

To make the cashew cream, drain the nuts and rinse well. Put all of the ingredients into a blender and pulse until smooth. Transfer to a small bowl and place in the fridge.

To make the taco filling, place all of the ingredients in a food processor and pulse until they have a texture like minced meat.

Wash and pat dry the lettuce leaves. Divide the avocado slices and the taco mix among the lettuce leaves and drizzle with the cashew cream. Serve with fresh lime wedges.

beet and fennel burgers on portobello buns

Who doesn't love a burger? As tasty as the Happy Cow Burgers (page 180) are, you don't always have to go for the meat option. This veggie-based recipe uses beetroot to give the hearty oompf that you expect from any decent burger. And because they pack in beetroot, onion and fennel – all excellent sources of fibre – these burgers give our gut microbes something to smile about. Instead of white refined buns I use portobello mushrooms, which give depth of flavour as well as a nutritional boost. Add some smashed avocado and a flourish of spinach leaves, which provide many of the nutrients we need for a healthy brain and gut, and this dish puts a whole new spin on mindful eating.

serves 2 (makes approx. 4 burgers)

½ small bulb fennel, trimmed and outer layer removed, cut into chunks

1 small beetroot, peeled and cut into chunks

¼ red onion, peeled and chopped

50g ground almonds

25g coconut flour

3 tablespoons ground flaxseed

25g activated walnuts (page 16)

1 teaspoon ground cumin

1 teaspoon mild smoked paprika

½ teaspoon mineral-rich salt

Generous pinch black pepper

1 organic free range egg, beaten

mushroom 'buns'

4 large portobello mushroom cups

Melted ghee or organic unsalted butter

2 teaspoons fresh thyme

Generous handful baby spinach leaves

avocado mash

1 avocado

Pinch mineral-rich salt

Preheat the oven to 200°C/Gas 6 and line two baking trays with baking parchment.

Prepare the mushroom buns by lightly brushing with melted ghee or butter, then place them on one of the trays.

Put the fennel, beetroot and onion into a food processor and pulse until finely chopped. Add the ground almonds, coconut flour, ground flaxseed, walnuts, cumin, paprika, salt and pepper to the processor. Add the egg and process until fully combined.

Take tennis ball-sized pieces of the beetroot mixture and flatten into burgers. Place them on the other lined baking tray and bake in the oven for 35 minutes. After about 15 minutes, put the mushrooms in the oven, so they have 20 minutes to bake.

Meanwhile, remove the flesh from the avocado and, using a fork, mash together with a generous pinch of salt.

To assemble, remove the mushroom 'buns' from the oven and sprinkle each of them with ½ teaspoon of fresh thyme leaves. Divide the avocado mash among the mushroom 'buns' and then place a few baby spinach leaves on each bone. Finally place the burgers on top.

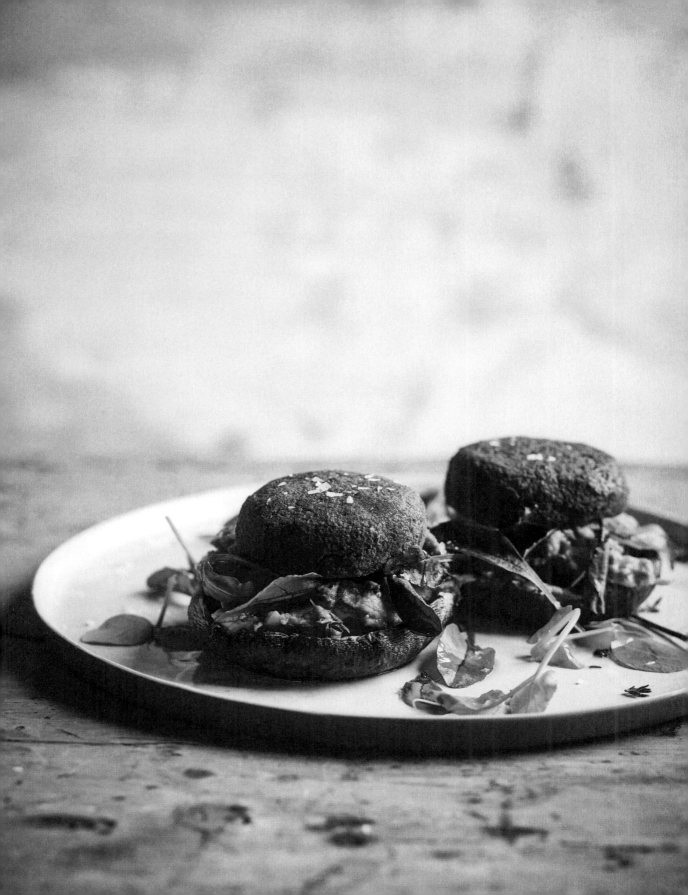

karma krackers

Shop-bought crackers can be seemingly healthy foods but they often provide little or no nutritional value or have ingredients that can leave your gut feeling less than happy. These crackers are designed to leave you feeling calmer and more balanced. This is down to the blend of soothing spices such as fennel and fenugreek; they also include flaxseed, which helps the bowels to move regularly and gently. These are great to serve with soups, and I think they go really well with my Shiitake, Leek and Seaweed Broth (you can see them alongside this recipe on page 205). Alternatively, for a savoury breakfast, why not try them with a generous spoonful of Spicy Carrot and Almond Spread (page 245) and a boiled egg.

makes 15 crackers

20g ground flaxseed
75g ground almonds
2 tablespoons hemp seeds
2 tablespoons sunflower seeds
¼ teaspoon garlic powder
1 teaspoon cumin seeds
1 teaspoon fennel seeds
½ teaspoon ground fenugreek
½ teaspoon ground turmeric
¼ teaspoon bicarbonate of soda
½ teaspoon mineral-rich salt
Generous pinch black pepper
1 tablespoon apple cider vinegar

Preheat the oven to 180°C/Gas 4. Place all of the dry ingredients in a large mixing bowl and mix thoroughly. Add the vinegar, then gradually add 60ml of filtered water – you may not need all of the water so go slow. Mix well and knead to form a dough.

Place the dough on a sheet of baking parchment and cover with another sheet. Use a rolling pin to roll out the dough to about 4mm thick.

Transfer carefully on to a baking tray and then remove the top layer of parchment. Score through the dough carefully with a knife to create 5cm-square crackers. Bake for 25 minutes. Carefully transfer to a wire rack and leave to cool fully before breaking into squares. Store in an airtight container. These should keep fresh for up to 2 weeks.

turmeric chai latte

This latte works well for a mid-afternoon boost rather than reaching for a coffee. Save your cup of joe for the morning, when it's much better for your stress hormones and sleep. This latte gives your brain and gut a boost just as much as a hit of caffeine. That's because it contains turmeric to help get those neurons firing and keep your gut on an even keel. It also contains maca powder, which helps the body to manage stress hormones and provides fibre for your gut microbes so they can produce plenty of the positive hormone serotonin. Savour and enjoy this and create your own oasis of calm.

serves 1

200ml Brazil nut milk (page 150), another nut milk, or raw or organic unhomogenised ful fat dairy milk

1 heaped teaspoon ground turmeric

½ teaspoon ground cinnamon

¼ teaspoon ground ginger

Generous pinch ground cardamom

Generous pinch black pepper

2 teaspoons maca powder

1 teaspoon coconut oil

Blend all the ingredients together in a high-speed blender. Pour into a small saucepan and heat gently for 2–3 minutes. Transfer to your favourite mug and sip gently.

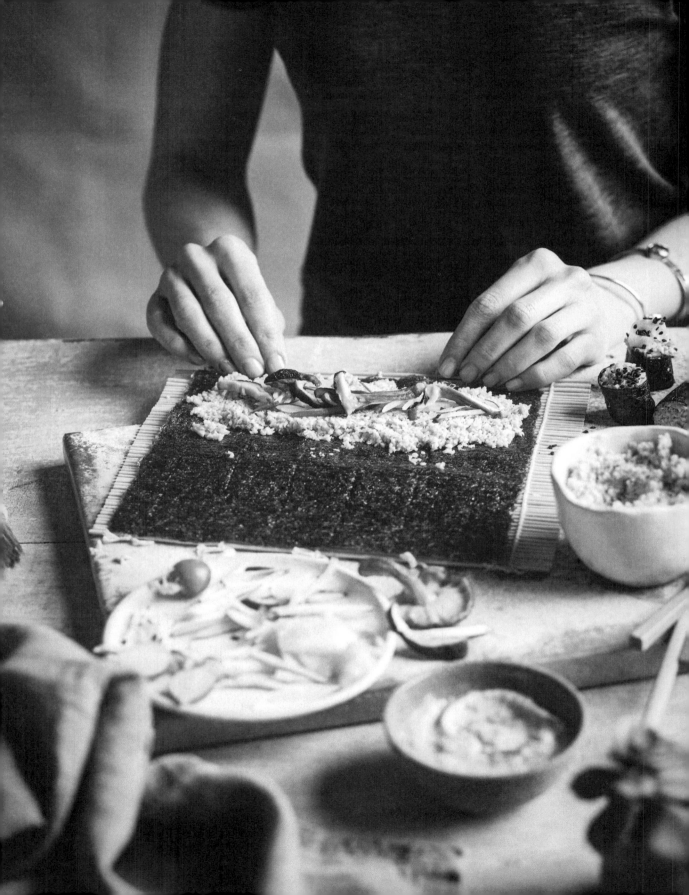

CHAPTER 9

on a hormonal trip

WHEN JAMES BROWN wrote 'Sex Machine' I'm pretty sure he didn't expect it to be mentioned in a book about the gut. But when it comes to being in tune with your sexy side, your digestive system plays a big part in how your hormones behave. The gut has a significant influence over our endocrine system, the glands that secrete hormones to manage and communicate a multitude of biochemical processes. In its own seductive way, the gut and its resident microbes exert authority over the body's metabolism and sex hormones, affecting fertility, sex drive, PMS and menopause, as well as managing hunger, appetite and weight. Indeed the gut is involved in many different hormonally related conditions that might be felt very far from the gut itself. In this chapter we'll explore these topics and learn how shaping the microbiome and supporting the gut can help us achieve a happy hormonal balance. To complement the information provided I've created recipes such as my glorious Wild Salmon with Roasted Carrots, Leaves and Miso Kefir Dressing (page 231), sumptuous Broccoli and Walnut Bread (page 226) and the brilliant Banana Miso Honey Crumble (page 232). You'll certainly be feeling much more positive – hormonally and otherwise – after making some of these lip-smacking recipes.

Let's start with what is probably the biggest cash cow when it comes to nutrition. Yes, I'm talking about the Holy Grail: the quest for weight loss. 'What is the magic formula?' I hear you cry. Well, first let's look at what hunger *really* means.

hunger games

Hunger is a weird thing. Sometimes it is a genuine feeling. Quite often it's not. Some of us are sensitive to even the slightest hint of hunger and find ourselves wanting to eat everything in sight. And then there are those who can go all day and say they 'forget to eat' – frankly, such people mystify me! Clearly the feeling of hunger is entirely subjective and often misinterpreted. For example, we may mistake thirst, boredom or stress for hunger. One thing is for sure: the gut has its own hormonal messengers that tell us when to eat and when we are full. So is the problem that we often choose not to listen to them? Or is it that somewhere along the line the communication channels are getting muddled?

I think it's fair to say that many of us have had that moment of staring into an open fridge, looking for answers to our problems, but rarely do we find them there. However, rather than beating ourselves up for succumbing to temptation, it may be reassuring to know that some of this behaviour is driven by hormones. In Chapter 1, I mentioned the hormones that kick-start certain digestive processes; when it comes to a rumbling tummy or recognising when you are full, again, a lot of it comes down to hormones.

Let's start with the feeling that you need to eat. This is driven by hormones such as neuropeptide Y, produced by the hypothalamus in the brain, and ghrelin, produced mainly by cells in the stomach. We'll discuss ghrelin in more detail in a second. Then there are hormones that help to curb the appetite. This is an extensive list that includes: peptide YY, which reduces appetite in response to

eating; cholecystokinin, one of the most widely investigated gut hormones, which helps to inhibit food intake; and glucagon-like peptide-1, which ensures a steady flow of nutrient absorption and enhances insulin secretion in order to balance blood sugar levels. One of the most important appetite regulators is leptin, which, unlike the above-mentioned hormones, is linked to longer-term regulation of energy balance rather than an immediate response to eating. Let's examine the pairing of ghrelin and leptin, dubbed our 'hunger hormones', in more detail.

feed me now

You might like to think of ghrelin as the 'feed me now' hormone: it is a fast-acting hormone that signals the body to eat. Leptin, 'the appetite suppressor', tells us to stop eating. These hormones are produced in the stomach, small intestine and adipose (fat) cells in response to insulin levels and body fat percentage, and they send their signals to the brain. At least, in a functioning gut–brain–hormone loop this is how it *should* work, but often the conversation gets disrupted. There are a couple of reasons for this. Firstly, bolting down our food in a nanosecond gives no time for leptin to kick in and say, 'Stop, we've had enough', so we just continue to eat and then suddenly feel stuffed. Sound familiar? This is another reason why chewing your food well is so important. Yes, I know I sound like a stuck record, but chewing properly has implications for weight management as it gives leptin enough time to let us know when we are full. One of the other reasons for this disrupted communication is 'leptin resistance', which means the body doesn't respond properly to the hormone's signals. Research has shown that many overweight or obese people are prone to this. In essence, they cannot tune in to the feeling of being satisfied.

But are there ways to influence these hormones and control our sometimes unruly and insatiable appetites? Yes there are but, funnily enough, they don't involve food.

ways to influence your hunger hormones

Get some decent sleep If you don't get enough shut-eye these hormones can shift out of balance. Conversely, regular good quality sleep decreases ghrelin levels, which means a reduced appetite. Ghrelin also increases our natural growth hormone, shifting body fat to lean muscle, and more muscle means a faster metabolism as muscle burns more calories than fat.

Drink more water Ghrelin isn't just about regulating our food intake; it's also about fluids. We often confuse hunger with thirst. Next time you think you are hungry between meals, try having a glass of water or herbal tea and see if that curbs the need to dive head-first into the biscuit tin.

Work out first thing in the morning This can help to support glucose tolerance for better and more balanced blood sugar management, so you might want to rethink your gym schedule.

Manage your stress level This is vital since increased stress, specifically the stress hormone cortisol, has been shown to increase ghrelin. That's why we typically gravitate to the fridge when we feel the pressures of life. See Chapter 8 for a discussion on stress and how to manage it.

what's the gut got to do with it?

Although these hormones are important when it comes to hunger and weight management, this isn't the full picture. The role of the microbiome has recently become a hot topic when it comes to people's ever-expanding waistlines.

The ratio of microbial species in the gut is a key factor. If you have made many failed attempts to lose weight you could be housing a naturally more 'obese' microbiome rather than one that is more 'lean' in its composition. This ratio is specifically linked with certain types of gut bacteria, namely *Bacteroidetes* and *Firmicutes*. It seems that the dominance of one or other of these will make you more or less predisposed to weight gain. Studies have found that the microbiomes of those who are naturally lean have higher numbers of *Bacteroidetes*, whereas those with a larger proportion of *Firmicutes* are more likely to be overweight.

Furthermore, it appears that not only does the ratio of gut bacteria leave some people with a greater propensity towards weight gain but the amount of calories that they extract from food is higher. While this might be a relatively small difference for each meal, the cumulative effect means it can soon add up. Since our gut bacteria influence how much energy each of us extracts from our food, it does somewhat put the kibosh on the whole notion of obsessive calorie counting.

On the plus side, studies show we can also shape the landscape of our microbiomes in response to the foods we eat, cultivating microbes that thrive on the foods we eat most regularly. Let's take sugar as an example: if you eat a lot of sugary foods then you will naturally support the growth of microbes that are efficient at absorbing sugar and can extract as many calories as possible so they also have a veritable feast. On the other hand, if you don't eat very much sugar then the species that dominate your microbiome won't necessarily absorb it as easily since they are not accustomed to it. This makes sense from an evolutionary perspective as our microbiome seeks optimum energy.

If you also have a more 'obese' microbiome, then the fat storage genes may get switched on more frequently, which is partly why some people continually struggle to lose weight.

As well as helping to determine how much energy we extract from what we eat, your microbiome also has a significant influence on how your body uses that energy – either utilising it immediately for fuel, or storing it as fat tissue. Bacteria can switch genes on and off to signal when to store or use energy. This makes sense for their own survival: your gut provides a cosy home for them, so it's in their interests to make sure you have a supply of energy to get through the 'tough times'. If you also have a more 'obese' microbiome, then the fat storage genes may get switched on more frequently, which is partly why some people continually struggle to lose weight, despite trying every diet under the sun. It really isn't a straightforward equation of the energy you take in versus how much of it you burn.

Before we leave the weight debate we also need to look at the possible connection between intestinal permeability aka leaky gut, obesity and type 2 diabetes. In Chapter 4 we looked at leaky gut, whereby the barrier of the gut can become compromised and more permeable, allowing unwarranted substances to pass through into the bloodstream. Among these substances are lipopolysaccharides (LPSs). When they escape the confines of the gut and enter the bloodstream they can set off a cascade of inflammatory responses in the immune system. This inflammatory 'alarm bell' is thought to also affect our fat storage cells, causing them to increase in size. Therefore one might even consider overweight and obese people to be in a chronic state of low level inflammation. Increased circulating lipopolysaccharides may also disrupt the production of insulin, which can lead to insulin resistance and, potentially, type 2 diabetes. You can see how there is a real domino effect when the gut is out of whack – and that has implications for the number on the scales, too.

If you want to achieve a more svelte physique then you need to support a leaner microbiome, as well as a robust gut barrier, by giving the gut and your 'lean' microbes all the nutrients they need to survive and thrive. (See Chapter 4 for more on helping to restore a leaky gut or start with the Weed, Seed and Feed programme on page 46.) The way that we extract energy from our food and store it is guided by the dynamics in the gut and fundamentally relies on nourishing the microbiome. Eating plenty of the right types of fibre, natural probiotics and prebiotics – which we covered in Chapter 2 – is essential to support the growth of beneficial bacteria. Choosing good quality sources of fat can also help to prevent piling on the pounds. Yes, that does include butter! (See box opposite)

butter is back!

Butter and its cousin ghee (clarified butter) have been around for millennia and for good reason. In recent decades, butter has been swerved by fat phobics and calorie counters due to its high levels of saturated fat. But consuming saturated fat doesn't always mean moving up a dress size. It can actually have the opposite effect, as the right types of dietary fat help to support metabolic processes and provide vital nutrients that, in turn, lead to a healthy weight. Rather than avoiding butter you need to be more cautious about having too many refined processed foods and sugar.

Margarine is one of the most highly processed foods, and is often made from hydrogenated polyunsaturated oils that have damaging effects on our health, due to the altered chemical structure of the fats it contains. These oils can be difficult for us to excrete and create increased oxidisation and inflammation in the body, which is linked to an increased risk of cardiovascular disease, diabetes and digestive issues. Similar oils are used in many other processed foods, such as pies, cakes and biscuits, and in many fried foods.

In contrast, naturally occurring compounds in butter such as conjugated linolenic acid and butyrate have anti-inflammatory properties and other protective benefits. We also need the types of saturated fat found in butter for optimum hormone balance and neurotransmitter functioning. If you restrict them too much you are likely to feel pretty miserable and hungry as they also help to provide satiety and stabilise blood sugar levels.

Butter is also a great source of pre-formed vitamin A (the kind that is more easily absorbed by the body), and it contains vitamins D and E too. Finally vitamin K_2 in butter from grass-fed cows can have significant benefits when it comes to maintaining strong bones and reducing the risk of cardiovascular disease. Of course this doesn't mean you should be slicing it off in great chunks, but used moderately butter certainly has a place in your diet. Always opt for the grass-fed organic and unsalted kind to get the full benefits. And because butter has a high smoke point it's one of the better fats for cooking at high temperatures; leave the cold pressed oils to drizzle over your cooked food. Hurrah for butter and all of its benefits!

the gas pedal

Let's return to the relationship between our hormones and the gut and, more specifically, an intricate organ called the thyroid that works a bit like a thermostat for the body's metabolism. You might equate the thyroid to the accelerator in a car. If you step on the pedal it speeds things up; ease off and it slows down. The same is true for how the thyroid affects the entire body, including the gut.

So, what are the symptoms of a thyroid whose speedometer is faulty? Well, perhaps your get up and go has gone, or you have an increased sensitivity to the cold, constipation, menstrual problems, dry skin or weight gain. These can all be signs of an underactive thyroid, or hypothyroidism. Conversely, an

overproduction of thyroid hormones –
hyperthyroidism – can lead to symptoms
such as heart palpitations, insomnia, more
frequent bowel movements and increased
sweating. However, for those suffering with
thyroid issues it is generally more common
that there is not enough fuel in the tank.
And this has a lot to do with the gut.

hypothyroidism and the gut

The gut can affect the thyroid in a couple of
ways. Firstly, because our gut bacteria play
a significant role in how active our thyroid
hormones are, a compromised microbiome
can slow things down (we'll come onto that
shortly). However, it isn't simply about how
well – or otherwise – our microbes convert
hormones; it is also strongly linked with
the health of the gut barrier. As we saw in
Chapter 4, if bacteria or food molecules
escape the confines of the gut and find their
way into the bloodstream, this can elicit an
immune response. If the response is sustained,
it can result in an overactive immune system
and may be one of the possible factors in the
development of some autoimmune conditions,
where 'innocent' tissue gets caught in the
crossfire. The same is true with the thyroid
and can result in an autoimmune-driven
condition called Hashimoto's thyroiditis, in
which the immune system mistakenly destroys
thyroid tissue along with its ability
to function.

However, this is not where the story ends.
Thyroid hormones are partly responsible for
keeping the gut lining robust, and preventing
substances from getting out of bounds in the
first place. Indeed, if the thyroid hormones
T3 and T4 are low then this can affect the

Good quality sources of fibre
not only feed and bolster the
microbiome but also get the
bowels moving.

protective lining of the gut and lead to increased
intestinal permeability. It's a vicious circle.
Other hormones, such as thyroid-stimulating
hormone and thyroid-releasing hormone,
also help to manage the gut's protective tissue
(GALT, or gut-associated lymphoid tissue),
which maintains the integrity of the gut
barrier. Moreover, with a more permeable
barrier comes the associated inflammatory
substances, lipopolysaccharides, which circulate
in the bloodstream and can impact on the
thyroid by decreasing thyroid hormone levels.
In short, a leaky gut can slow the pace of the
body's metabolism. It is very much a two-way
relationship between the gut and the thyroid.

Digging a little deeper, it turns out that our
gut bacteria help to convert the inactive form
of the thyroid hormone T4 into its active
counterpart T3, which keeps the metabolism
ticking along nicely. They do this by producing
an enzyme called intestinal sulfatase; in fact,
they create almost 20 per cent of the active
hormone, so you might think of this as a gut–
bacteria–thyroid *ménage à trois*. A compromised
microbiome can therefore significantly impair
this crucial conversion, so leaky gut or not
your thyroid can struggle if you don't have a
healthy microbiome. The thyroid may be the
accelerator, but once again the gut is well and
truly in the driving seat!

So, what should you do if you think you
may have a sluggish thyroid? Naturally you
have to begin by supporting the microbiome,

which also means identifying any food or other triggers that might be contributing to a compromised gut. In Chapter 4 we examined the connection between intestinal permeability and autoimmune disease, so, in a case of Hashimoto's hypothyroidism, it might be worth using similar strategies. Gluten in particular has been proposed as a potential food trigger associated with this, so going gluten free while supporting the microbiome and health of the gut barrier could be considered. However, I would urge you to consult a nutritional practitioner first, if you have been diagnosed with this condition.

It is also imperative to work on boosting beneficial bacteria to increase the conversion of thyroid hormones. Eating plenty of probiotic foods such as unpasteurised kimchi, sauerkraut, cheese and kefir will do this. Nutrients that nourish the gut barrier are also important (bone broth is a superstar for this because of its amino acid profile). So too are good quality sources of fibre, not just to feed and bolster the microbiome but also to get the bowels moving, as a sluggish gut can often be one of the main symptoms of hypothyroidism.

Other thyroid-supportive nutrients include magnesium – found in leafy green vegetables, avocados, nuts, seeds and sprouted grains – and selenium, of which you can get a good quota from just two Brazil nuts per day. But the most important thyroid nutrient is iodine, which is vital for the production of thyroid hormones. It is found in fish and shellfish, but the richest source is seaweed. Before you grimace at the thought, see the box on this page, which outlines why seaweed is so brilliant and how you can enhance the flavour of many a dish with a touch of algae.

seaweeds

Edible seaweeds have been used for centuries in the cuisines of China, Korea and Japan. They are more familiar to us in the form of nori, used to wrap sushi rolls (have a look at my Parsnip, Shiitake and Radish Sushi on page 229), and wakame, which is often added to miso soup. Seaweeds also feature in traditional dishes in some parts of the British Isles: laver bread in Wales and dulse in Ireland, for example.

Seaweed has been a buzzword on the trendy food scene for quite a while now, but what can this funky-looking algae do for our health and wellbeing?

Packed full of nutrients such as vitamins A and C and a decent source of calcium, seaweed's most potent mineral is iodine, which is crucial for regulating thyroid function. As with most things, too much iodine can have negative side effects, but as many of us are deficient in this vital mineral, seaweed is a natural way to boost your intake. Just make sure you get your seaweed from a supplier that harvests and sources it appropriately from clean water. See page 264 for my recommendation.

The question is then how to eat it? Try sprucing up a salad with dried seaweed, or adding it to scrambled eggs for a morning boost. I love adding seaweed to broths, such as the Shiitake, Leek and Seaweed Broth on page 204. It might be an acquired taste, but you'll soon be throwing it into all sorts of recipes.

let's talk about sex

You may have heard the expression 'food porn'; this is when we look at food and it creates a feeling akin to sexual euphoria. To be honest, seaweed is unlikely to have that effect (although my ice creams on pages 183–185 might), but when it comes to sexual arousal and satisfaction the gut has a strong influence on how we feel.

This is for all the ladies out there who have found themselves bloated like a balloon and obliged to cancel a social engagement or hot date because they can't fit into anything other than a tent.

You don't need me to point out that digestive symptoms such as gas, bloating, reflux and constipation are not ideal for creating a romantic ambience between the sheets. But there is another link between your gut and sexual feelings. Much of this is due to levels of serotonin in the body. This neurotransmitter, or chemical messenger, strongly influences our mood, and most of it is produced by bacteria in the gut. The reproductive organs are very sensitive to serotonin, so if the gut is not performing well then your sexual drive won't be up to much either. Having a healthy balance of hormones has a very strong correlation with our digestive health, too. Many hormonally related conditions, such as infertility and low libido, as well as female-specific conditions such as endometriosis and PCOS (polycystic ovarian syndrome), can be related to poor gut health. Let's look at this in a little more detail.

This is for all the ladies out there who have found themselves bloated like a balloon and obliged to cancel a social engagement or hot date because they can't fit into anything other than a tent. Usually we put this down to the time of the month or perhaps that we've been a bit slack with our food choices, but bloating may have less to do with what you are eating and more to do with what is going on with the bacteria in your gut.

If there is an imbalance in the microbiome this can lead directly to symptoms such as bloating and excess gas, neither of which is good for a night out on the town, but as we have seen throughout this book, the microbes in your gut don't simply affect digestive processes. In fact, when it comes to balancing hormones, they have a crucial role in metabolising oestrogen. Collectively these specialised bacteria have been referred to as the 'estrobolome' and if they are not doing their job efficiently then you may start to see symptoms of oestrogen dominance, such as PMS, mood swings, breast tenderness, hormone-related acne and a general loss of mojo. So those monthly meltdowns may have more to do with your gut than you think and by positively shifting your microbiome you could say goodbye to the inner beast that is often unleashed. The estrobolome has also been linked to conditions such as fibroids, endometriosis and polycystic ovaries. And before you chaps start to zone out and think this doesn't apply to you, it does. Oestrogen dominance in men is becoming a real issue with a series of negative health associations, including mood swings, poor muscle tone and gynecomastia (man boobs). Research is also linking this to an increased risk of prostate cancer. Other recent studies suggest that a variation in the estrobolome may increase the likelihood of developing oestrogen-related breast cancer in some women. Studies have suggested that this may go some way towards explaining why some people don't develop hormonally related cancers, despite having a genetic predisposition to do so. They just might have more efficient oestrogen-metabolising microbes and almost certainly a healthier gut.

How does this work? The microbes of the estrobolome use genetic codes to produce enzymes that work on metabolising, or removing, oestrogen in the gut. This happens in partnership with the liver and affects the amount of oestrogen circulating throughout the entire body. When there is also dysbiosis in the gut and not enough of these microbes to help support the process, the result can be a reabsorption of oestrogen, meaning it is not efficiently eliminated, and this adds a greater hormonal load to the system. So, as with hormone imbalance, it's important to also address the health of the gut and establish a microbiome that is diverse and plentiful so these metabolising microbes can work at their very best.

Getting your gut more hormonally in tune therefore comes back to nourishing it with the appropriate foods, such as probiotics, prebiotics and fibre. The Cinnamon Loaf on page 224 is packed with naturally sweet and comforting flavours but it also contains a wealth of these gut-soothing foods. It's a surefire way to get your gut and your hormones off to a very pleasant start to the day. And when it comes to hormonally supportive foods, cruciferous vegetables have got to be right up there. This is because one of the compounds they contain, Indole-3-carbinol (I3C), has been shown to have a profound effect on oestrogen metabolism. We're talking about vegetables such as

cauliflower, cabbage, kale, radish, turnip, the rather divisive Brussels sprout, and the powerhouse that is broccoli (see page 222).

maybe baby

One final hormone-related area where we regularly see strong correlations with gut health is fertility. I could write an entire book on the gut–fertility connection, but in the context of this book we can merely scratch the surface. You may not have even considered there is a connection at all, but the gut plays an important role in making babies.

Many clients come to me because although they can't seem to conceive, they have been told that there is 'nothing really wrong'. Nothing, that is, until we start talking about their gut health. If you are struggling to conceive then your gut could be one of the factors you need to consider. Let me explain why.

Firstly we need to look at how the microbiome, and more specifically the estrobolome, is performing. This is because our hormones are dependent on these microbes working hard to keep them in balance. Oestrogen-led symptoms such as PMS, mood swings and breast tenderness could indicate that your hormones are not in alignment and this can play a significant part in fertility.

It is also important to keep in mind that cortisol, one of our major stress hormones, can affect the ability to conceive. If your body is in a chronic state of fight or flight then your biological instinct is to survive, not procreate. Your body will not focus its resources on creating a child if it thinks that you are in danger.

broccoli

It probably comes as no surprise to find a section on broccoli in this book, but you might be taken aback by just how much health-boosting ammo this green machine contains.

Firstly there's the compound called Indole-3-carbinol (I3C). This is derived from a type of phytochemical present in cruciferous vegetables that becomes active when we chop or chew them. It plays a role in metabolising oestrogen in the body as well as supporting hormone detoxification pathways in the liver, which helps to stabilise overall hormone levels. Chewing broccoli also releases sulforaphane, which gives it its distinct 'sulphurous' taste and smell. This compound supports healthy cell turnover and natural detoxification processes. Studies have shown that these same compounds can also arrest the development of unhealthy cells, meaning they can potentially inhibit the development of tumours.

Pretty amazing stuff! But that's not where it ends. Our gut microbes like good quality fibre and broccoli provides this in abundance. Additionally, some of the active chemical compounds in broccoli help support microbial activity and work as natural antibiotics against certain pathogenic bacteria.

And let's not forget that broccoli is also an excellent source of vitamins and minerals, including: vitamin K, which is important for our bones and cardiovascular health; vitamin C to protect our cells from damage; chromium, which helps to balance blood sugar levels; and a wealth of B vitamins that have a role in energy production and many other vital processes, including balancing our hormones.

When it comes to getting it into your diet, broccoli sprouts pack the biggest punch and are a delicious way to top a salad. But whether it's tenderstem, purple sprouting or just your regular green variety it's fair to say that broccoli has earned its status as the pin-up of healthy foods. One final tip: if you want to maximise the effect of some of the compounds in broccoli, combine it with a touch of strong mustard powder. Make an olive oil and apple cider vinaigrette with a pinch of mustard powder to drizzle over it – delicious. My Broccoli and Walnut Bread (page 226) also uses this combo and it's something you can make ahead (or freeze), so you can make it a regular part of your routine. My Miso Cod with Wasabi Broccoli (page 34) has a similar nutrition-boosting effect.

While external stress is indeed a significant factor for fertility and must be addressed with *daily* pockets of recovery, such as breathing exercises, gentle yoga or even simply eating your meals in a relaxing environment, much of the overall stress load may come internally from a gut that is struggling. This includes chronic gut infections that compromise the absorption of crucial nutrients needed to support a more fertile environment. A gut with an imbalanced microbiome can also put the body into a persistent state of inflammation, which also creates ongoing stress.

The link between stress and fertility is equally important for men. Low sperm count or slow-moving sperm can be related to being under too much stress.

When it comes to fertility, it's not just the microbes in the gut that play a role. The vagina has its own microbiome and it is vital that this is kept at the right pH level (slightly acidic) to prevent an overgrowth of troublesome bacteria. Negative shifts in the vaginal microbiome can also create infections and low grade inflammation that can impact on fertility. Encouraging the growth of beneficial bacteria is also very important during pregnancy. As we saw in Chapter 2, these microbes will be passed on to the newborn child during a natural birth, so a healthy and diverse population will help support a robust immune system and a healthy gut right from the get go. A strong microbiome is possibly the best head start you can give your new bundle of joy and that's exactly how Mother Nature intended it to be. The Weed, Seed and Feed programme on page 46 can help you to start to achieve balance and nourish your own fertile 'garden'. But I would advise working directly with a registered practitioner if this is your goal.

keeping your hormones happy

It may have surprised you to discover that the gut and its multitude of microbes play such an important role in how your hormones behave. I bet you never imagined that nourishing your gut could help you to achieve a consistent weight and potentially be part of the journey towards starting a family. Of course when it comes to hormonal health there are other factors to consider, but nourishing the gut certainly has a place in keeping your hormones balanced and happy. And with some of the recipes that follow, such as my comforting Cinnamon and Thyme French Sourdough Toast (page 227) or my Banana Miso Honey Crumble (page 232), this can be a sweetly inspired hormonal trip too.

cinnamon loaf

This sumptuous loaf is based on chestnut flour, which is brimming with gut-friendly fibre, and almonds, which are an excellent prebiotic food. But the real hero ingredient is warming cinnamon, one of the best sources of chromium, which helps to balance blood sugar levels and our hunger hormones. Cinnamon also blends perfectly with the chestnut flour and almonds to provide our gut microbes with a sweet feast. Because this uses chia seeds to bind, it's great for those who don't do so well with eggs or are following a vegan diet. Serve it with some sliced banana or with a generous spoonful of coconut kefir. It's great for breakfast and you can make it in advance and freeze it if you want to. It will keep for up to 5 days in the fridge.

makes 1 loaf

2 tablespoons chia seeds

120ml warm filtered water

80g chestnut flour

100g ground almonds

45g flaked almonds

4 tablespoons coconut flour

45g activated pecans (page 16)

1 teaspoon bicarbonate of soda

1 tablespoon ground cinnamon

2 tablespoons almond nut butter

2 tablespoons coconut oil, plus extra for greasing

2 tablespoons apple cider vinegar

Seeds from 1 vanilla pod

200ml unsweetened almond milk

Preheat the oven to 150°C/Gas 2. Line a 23 x 12cm loaf tin with baking parchment and grease with a small amount of coconut oil.

Mix the chia seeds with the water in a small bowl and set aside.

Place all the remaining ingredients, except the almond milk, in a food processor and pulse to combine. Then add the chia mixture and the almond milk and pulse again to get a sticky cake mixture. Spoon this into the loaf tin and level the top. Bake for 1 hour, then check that it's done by turning out and tapping the bottom: it should sound hollow. If not, return it to the oven for 5–10 minutes. Turn out onto a wire rack and leave to cool completely before slicing.

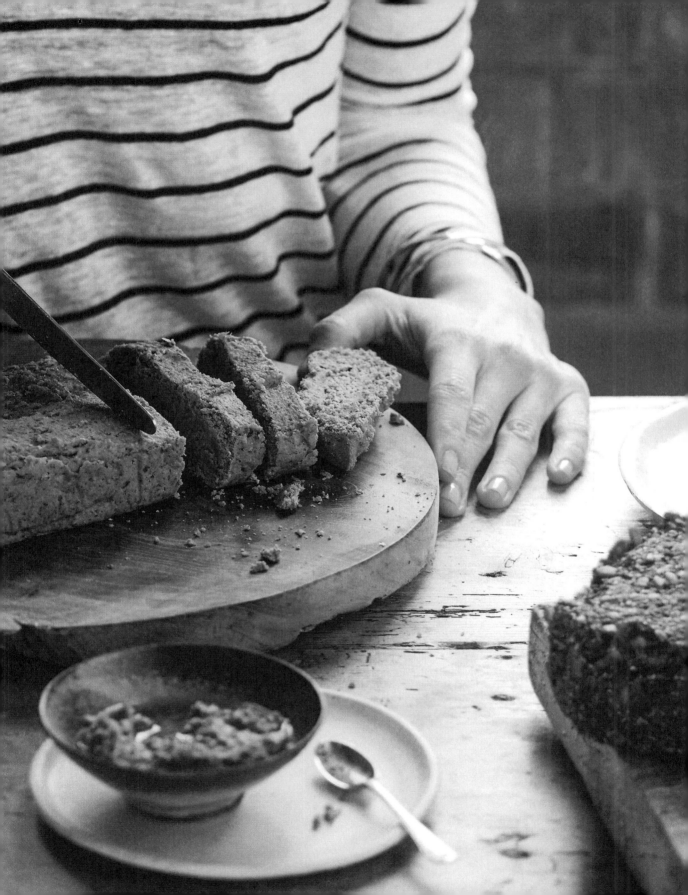

broccoli and walnut bread

Broccoli gained its reputation as a nutritional powerhouse for a multitude of reasons: one of the compounds it contains supports the metabolism of hormones such as oestrogen. This green machine also contains sulforaphane, which can have a positive effect on the immune system as well as supporting the beneficial microbes in the gut. The mustard powder helps to make those positive chemicals in the broccoli more readily available to the body. Science aside, broccoli is an awesome base for this bread. It's brilliant as an open sandwich with tinned sardines and some pesto, such as my Watercress Pesto (page 28). It also makes a delicious accompaniment to soups or for breakfast with a couple of poached eggs. Keep it wrapped in the fridge for up to 5 days, or freeze it. Perfect for a Sunday afternoon of baking to make your bread for the week ahead.

makes 1 loaf

1 very large head broccoli or 2 small ones

50g activated walnuts (page 16)

50g ground almonds

2 large organic free range eggs

4 tablespoons ground flaxseed

2 tablespoons nutritional yeast flakes

2 tablespoons apple cider vinegar

½ teaspoon bicarbonate of soda

½ teaspoon mineral-rich salt

Generous pinch black pepper

1 teaspoon yellow mustard powder

1 tablespoon finely chopped fresh sage

2 teaspoons dried or fresh marjoram

Preheat the oven to 180°C/Gas 4. Line a 23 x 12cm loaf tin with baking parchment so that it hangs over the sides.

Cut the broccoli into smaller florets and pulse in a food processor until you have a fine, rice-like texture. Add all of the remaining ingredients and pulse until evenly mixed. Spoon this carefully into the loaf tin and level the top with the back of a metal spoon. Bake for 40–45 minutes.

Lift up the baking parchment to remove the loaf and place it on a wire rack. Leave to cool completely before slicing.

cinnamon and thyme french sourdough toast

French toast is one of those dishes that invokes a feeling of comfort and joy whenever I eat it. My recipe uses sourdough because its process of fermentation naturally makes it a more digestive-friendly option than some other breads. The star ingredient here is the ghee or butter: both contain healthy saturated fats that are important in keeping our hormones balanced as well as supporting digestion. Enjoy this simple and glorious breakfast with Labneh (see page 64) or Coconut Vanilla Kefir (see page 81). For extra decadence and another gut-friendly boost, pair with some whipped raw dairy cream. *Bon appetit!*

serves 2

1 organic free range egg

50ml milk (I use raw dairy milk but you can use organic unhomogenised full fat dairy milk; unsweetened cashew milk works well too)

Seeds from 1 vanilla pod

2 tablespoons ghee or organic unsalted butter, plus extra for cooking

1 teaspoon ground cinnamon, plus a little extra for dusting

1 teaspoon roughly chopped fresh thyme

2–4 slices sourdough (depending on size)

Generous handful of blueberries

Crack the egg into a bowl and whisk together with the milk and vanilla.

In a small bowl, combine the ghee or butter with the cinnamon and thyme, then heat gently in a small saucepan on a low heat. Put to one side.

Heat a little extra ghee or butter in a frying pan on a medium heat. Dip the sourdough into the egg mix, turning to coat both sides evenly, then cook on one side for 3 minutes. Flip and cook on the other side for a further 3 minutes.

Lay the French toast on two plates and drizzle the cinnamon butter evenly over the slices. Dust with extra cinnamon and serve with blueberries.

thai coconut and butternut noodle broth

This veggie-based soup not only packs in flavour but is also super-soothing for the gut. This comes from the bone broth base that includes essential amino acids as well as coconut milk, which together help to soothe and support the health of the gut barrier.

serves 2 (with extra thai paste)

thai paste

2 teaspoons ground ginger

4 teaspoons ground cumin

4 teaspoons ground coriander

½–1 teaspoon chilli flakes

2 teaspoons galangal

¼ teaspoon garlic powder

4 teaspoons onion powder

Juice of 2 limes

4 tablespoons coconut aminos

4 tablespoons tomato paste

Couple pinches mineral-rich salt

½ tablespoon coconut oil

500ml Chicken Bone Broth (see page 57) (replace with vegetable stock for vegan version)

200ml full fat coconut milk

1 medium butternut squash, peeled and seeded, put through a spiraliser to make 'noodles'

2 medium carrots, peeled and cut into thin batons

2 pak choi, trimmed

2 spring onions, sliced thinly

Generous handful fresh coriander, roughly chopped (plus a few extra whole leaves to garnish)

1 tablespoon crushed cashews to garnish

Place all the ingredients for the paste in a small bowl and mix thoroughly. Transfer into a container as you will have extra to use for another supper.

In a large saucepan heat the coconut oil on a medium heat. Add 4 tablespoons of the paste and cook for 3 minutes. Add the bone broth and coconut milk and cook on a gentle simmer for 5 minutes. Add the butternut squash 'noodles' and carrots and simmer for another 5 minutes. Add the pak choi and spring onions and simmer for another 3 minutes. Remove the pan from the heat. Add the fresh coriander and stir to combine.

Divide between two bowls, add a touch more coriander and the crushed cashews to garnish.

parsnip, shiitake and radish sushi

Sushi might seem complicated to make but it's actually really simple. All you need is a sushi mat and you're away. I have used parsnips to create the 'rice' because they nourish our gut microbes and give exceptional depth of flavour. They work particularly well with the addition of coconut aminos, an alternative to soy sauce that has a naturally sweet, sticky and salty taste. Just like traditional sushi my version (see page 212) uses nori sheets: this nutrient-dense algae allows the beneficial bacteria in the gut to flourish and gives an iodine boost for the thyroid, which manages the body's metabolism. Add prebiotic mushrooms and gut-friendly radishes and this is sushi like you have never tasted before.

serves 1 generously or 2 as a side or starter

1 teaspoon coconut oil

6 shiitake mushrooms (or button or other mushrooms if you prefer), thinly sliced

4 radishes

2 nori sheets

parsnip 'rice'

2 parsnips, peeled and roughly chopped

½ tablespoon coconut aminos

¼ teaspoon garlic powder

1 tablespoon cashew nut butter

Pinch mineral-rich salt

wasabi cream

30g activated cashews (page 16)

50ml filtered water

1 teaspoon mirin

Wasabi powder (start with ¼ teaspoon and increase to your desired taste – it's hot!)

to garnish

Sprinkling black sesame seeds

Pickled ginger slices

Tamari

To make the wasabi cream, put all of the ingredients into a high-speed blender and pulse until thick and creamy. You may need to stop and scrape. Transfer to a small glass or ceramic bowl and place in the fridge. It will keep, covered, for up to 2 days.

To make the parsnip rice, place all of the ingredients in a food processor and pulse until you have a sticky rice-like texture. Place to one side.

Heat the coconut oil in a shallow pan, add the mushrooms and lightly stir-fry until just tender. Place in a small bowl and leave to cool. While they are cooling, slice the radishes into matchsticks.

Lay out a nori sheet on a sushi mat. On the nearest end spread half the parsnip rice so it covers a third of the sheet. Layer half of the radish slices and half of the cooked mushrooms lengthwise along the middle of the parsnip rice. Using the sushi mat, roll the nori away from you. Once you get to the end, moisten the edge of the nori sheet so that it sticks to itself. Turn the nori roll and using a very sharp knife cut into about eight smaller pieces. Repeat with the other sheet.

Garnish each with a sprinkling of black sesame seeds, a small piece of pickled ginger and a couple of drops of tamari. Serve with a couple of teaspoons of the wasabi cream on the side to dip your rolls into. Best eaten with chopsticks!

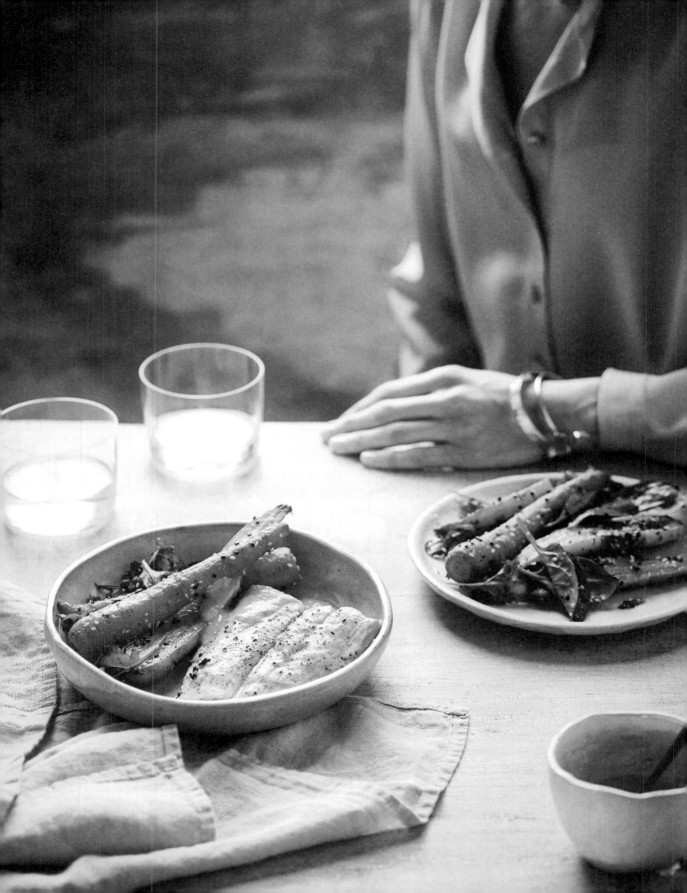

wild salmon with roasted carrots, leaves and miso kefir

Wild salmon has a distinctive vibrant orange colour and is typically higher in anti-inflammatory omega 3 essential fatty acids than farmed salmon, so it is best to buy this if it is available. The miso kefir dressing is packed full of natural probiotics that give a delicious boost to the gut and it's super-easy to make. Paired with buttery carrots this recipe is comfort food, gut-friendly style.

serves 2

6–8 carrots in various colours

4 tablespoons melted ghee or unsalted organic butter

Generous pinch mineral-rich salt

2 wild salmon fillets, approx. 135g each

miso kefir

2 tablespoons unpasteurised miso paste

2 tablespoons dairy kefir

Dash of sesame oil

Generous handful baby spinach or other seasonal leaves

3 tablespoons sesame seeds

Preheat the oven to 200°C/Gas 6.

Thoroughly wash your carrots and pat dry but don't peel them as there is a lot of nutrition in the skin. You can leave the tops on or trim them down if they are very long. Place in a roasting tray or an ovenproof dish, drizzle with the melted ghee or butter and sprinkle with salt. Cover with foil and place in the oven for 30–40 minutes until tender. Remove the foil and cook for a further 10 minutes.

While the carrots are cooking, lightly season the salmon fillets and place them on a baking tray lined with baking parchment. When you remove the foil from the carrots, pop the salmon in the oven; it should take 10 minutes to cook.

While the salmon is cooking, prepare the dressing by mixing the miso paste, kefir and sesame oil together; place to one side.

Once the salmon and the carrots are cooked, transfer the carrots to a large bowl, add the leaves and the sesame seeds. Stir well to combine, so the leaves begin to wilt. Divide the carrots between the plates and drizzle with the miso kefir dressing and finally add the salmon.

banana miso honey crumble

You might think of banana and miso as a somewhat unusual flavour combo but they work harmoniously together in this delicious crumble. This pairing combines both prebiotic and probiotic foods that support the balance of the microbiome, so from a gut perspective this dish gets a resounding thumbs-up. A touch of raw honey gives another gut boost and with the crunchy crumble becomes a total joy to eat. It's great for dessert, breakfast or you might like to halve the serving and enjoy it as a mid-afternoon treat. I like to serve it topped with physalis or other berries as they give a nice contrast of flavour.

serves 4

banana miso cream

65g cashews, soaked for 2 hours
2 unripe bananas
2 tablespoons sweet white miso paste
40g desiccated coconut
4 tablespoons unsweetened coconut yogurt
1 tablespoon raw honey
1 teaspoon ground ginger
1 teaspoon ground cinnamon

crumble

50g ground almonds
90g flaked almonds
20g coconut chips
2 tablespoons coconut flour
2 tablespoons raw honey
1 tablespoon melted coconut oil
1 teaspoon ground cinnamon
Pinch mineral-rich salt

Preheat the oven to 180°C/Gas 4. Line a baking sheet with baking parchment.

To make the crumble, place all the ingredients in a large bowl and mix together until you get a crumble-like texture. Place on the baking sheet and bake for 25 minutes, stirring after 15 minutes to toast evenly.

While this is cooking, make your banana miso cream. Drain the cashews and rinse thoroughly. Put all of the ingredients into a high-speed blender and pulse on a high setting until smooth. Transfer to a glass or ceramic bowl and put in the fridge.

Once the crumble is cooked, leave to cool for at least 10 minutes before assembling.

In four glasses or small bowls, start with a layer of the crumble (2–3 tablespoons), then a layer of the banana cream (2–3 tablespoons), another layer of the crumble and the banana cream, and finally a sprinkling of the crumble.

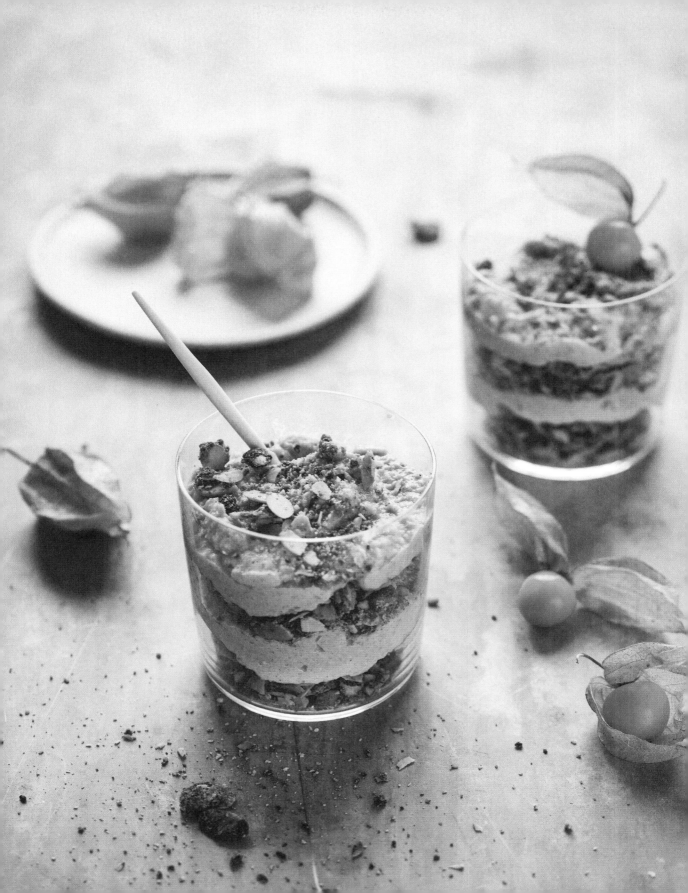

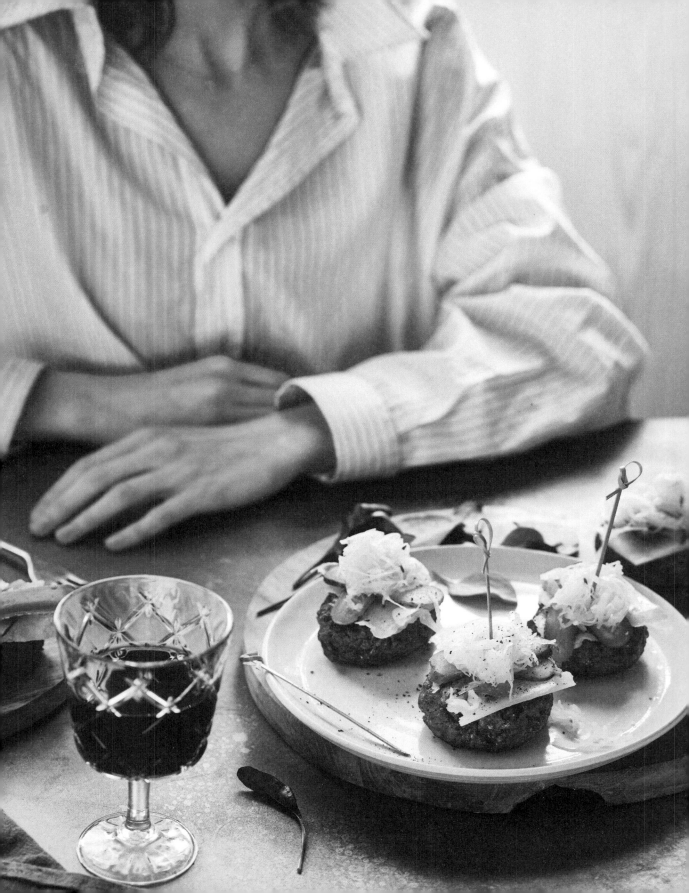

10

truth and lies

NUTRITION IS A baffling subject. One minute we're encouraged to follow the most in vogue diet or detox and then along comes an entirely contradictory regime that is said to be the next big thing. It's easy to be tempted to invest in a fancy supplement or powder that promises to be life-transforming or to be sucked into following the latest trend by glossy ad campaigns, beautiful endorsers and multiple social media images. But all this information can leave you feeling overwhelmed and confused.

In this chapter I will attempt to strip back a lot of the misconceptions and uninformed opinions behind some of the most popular trends and the outlandish advice that often goes with them. I'll demystify terms such as 'detox' and explain why the simplest approach to nutrition – no quick fixes or fads but honest, real food – is almost always the best way to nourish your body and your gut on a daily basis.

The recipes in this chapter champion tasty and wholesome dishes, such as my slow-cooked Harissa Lamb-Stuffed Cabbage Rolls (page 253) or the comforting Celeriac and Kraut Rösti (page 248). As you'll soon discover, food doesn't have to be complicated to be healthy; nor does it have to be devoid of flavour, flair and frivolity to be nutritious.

Let's start by looking at one of the most confusing and often misleading concepts out there. Yes, I'm talking about detoxing. Is it ridiculous nonsense? Or is there some logic behind this phenomenon?

detoxing: don't believe the hype

There is no doubt that the detox industry is booming. Most of us have at some point felt the desire to embark on a detox, typically in January in the aftermath of festive indulgence or at the prospect of getting into a swimsuit or sleeveless tee as summer looms. Manufacturers know that we are lured by the promise of gaining that elusive glow or svelte physique so they'll stick the word 'detox' on anything from a generic salad to a juice recipe, tea or supplement. And we, it seems, are hooked. After all, what's not to love? A detox promises not only to shift those surplus pounds but give you brighter skin, reduce troubling digestive symptoms and flush out all those pesky 'toxins' from of your system in a matter of days. But can detoxing really live up to the hype?

Firstly it is important to understand what the term detox means. From a medical perspective it refers to removing harmful and addictive substances such as poisons, drugs and alcohol from the body. More recently it has found a more mainstream definition as a short-term diet that involves abstinence from certain foods, often while following elaborate health and beauty regimes. The idea is that following such principles will cleanse the body of its general 'toxic overload'. Detoxes range from eliminating foods such as sugar, caffeine, alcohol and refined processed foods to excluding broader food groups, with dairy and gluten two of the most popular. There are also liquid fasting regimes as well as specific pills and products designed to 'aid' the process.

To be fair to the advocates of detoxing, the idea of abstinence isn't a new one. Our ancestors would embark on complete fasts to support the body's regenerative processes, and there is certainly research to back up this as a way to help decrease certain inflammatory markers, as long as it is used in a very targeted way. Note, however, that I said *complete* fasts. Fasting, specifically a type called 'time-restricted eating', in some individuals, may help support the diversity and activity of the microbiome. Time-restricted eating means consuming food only within a period of 9–12 hours and fasting for at least 12 hours between the last meal of the day and the first meal of the following day. Studies have shown this can also have a positive effect on weight management. However, the concept of targeted fasting is far removed from the modern pseudo-medical phenomenon of detoxing, which most people undertake in the hope of a quick route to a flatter stomach, rather than for the benefit of their microbes. Furthermore, most of these detox regimes fail to identify which 'toxins' are problematic, which leaves the whole principle open to even greater scepticism.

trust your body's own detox mechanism

Let's get down to the science of how the body detoxes. As we saw in Chapter 1, the body has its own highly developed and specially designed mechanisms for detoxifying and eliminating potentially harmful substances. The liver, kidneys, lungs, skin, enzymes and the gut and its many microbes work together like a well-oiled machine to get rid of toxins without causing any adverse effects. The concept that we build up an accumulation of waste or toxic products is, for the majority of us, simply not true. Of course many of us – particularly if we live in a polluted environment and have an unhealthy diet – are bombarded by substances from the air we breathe and the food we eat, but to say that the body needs to 'have a break' has no real merit as there is categorically no scientific evidence to back this up.

To compound the irony here, restricting food groups for longer periods of time may have the opposite effect from what you are trying to achieve because the body needs to ingest certain nutrients to enable the enzymes that are responsible for detoxification to do their job properly. The purported benefits of some of the more invasive (and frankly unpleasant) detox procedures, such as colonic irrigation, are also unsubstantiated and can cause more harm than good. The same goes for the overuse of laxative-type colon-cleansing tablets. Our gut bacteria don't like being flushed out and, crucially, this process gets shot of beneficial bacteria as well as the more pathogenic ones. Moreover, if you have any longstanding health conditions, continuing on any extreme regime can have detrimental knock-on effects. These kind of radical diets also fail to address the fact that we are all unique, so one person's natural detoxification processes may not be as efficient as another's. By their very nature, one-size-fits-all detox regimes cannot take into account factors such as underlying gut issues and/or the health of the microbiome, hormone imbalances, genetic predispositions and stress, all of which will have an impact on the outcome.

But detoxes aren't all bad. If you are someone who cannot curb your cravings, pressing the stop button on eating too much processed refined food, alcohol, caffeine and sugar has

why do some detoxes work?

It depends on your definition of success. Any kind of calorie-restrictive regime will help you drop a few pounds, but it is likely that the the weight loss will be short-lived. During a detox you lose mostly water and some stored glycogen (glucose used for energy) so as soon as you start to eat normally, you put this straight back on. If you continue any of these diets for a longer period it can have a detrimental effect on your metabolism by reducing your basal metabolic rate (the amount of energy expended when you are resting). The net result is that you end up with a slower metabolism than when you started.

got to be a good thing. For many people, doing a detox of this nature can mark a shift from negative eating patterns, binges and triggers, and that's important to recognise. If detoxing means 'cleansing the palate' – introducing more nutrient-dense whole foods and cutting down on white, fried and dyed foods – it can only be supportive. You can use my Weed, Seed and Feed programme on page 46 to help you on the road to a better long-term approach to this.

When it comes to alcohol, having alcohol-free days as part of your general lifestyle is certainly healthy but the idea that you need to go on a detox to cleanse your liver is a fallacy. In fact, drinking alcohol in small amounts regulates the enzymes needed to break it down, which also primes the liver to break down toxins in a more general sense. Plus, as we saw in Chapter 7, your gut can benefit from the occasional glass of wine.

Some of the basic actions I've looked at throughout this book, such as increasing your intake of clean water, getting good quality sleep and chewing your food thoroughly, will have much more of a long-term detoxing effect than any flash in the pan regime.

The most effective way to support natural detoxification processes is therefore to embrace a lifestyle that is balanced and not reactive, and that supports the health of the gut. Forget restrictive diets and instead be as inclusive as you possibly can while listening to what works for *your* body. If you tell yourself you cannot have something ever again, it will automatically invoke your inner rebel, so allow yourself to be free of too many rules – and that means having the odd treat now and then.

natural detox aids

Exercise is one of the best ways to support natural detoxification, and the gut loves moving too, so get outdoors and walk or run, book that yoga class, have a go at boxing or even put on your favourite music and rock out in your living room (a friend calls this her 'domestic disco'). Whatever gets you moving is good and it also gets you away from the endless stream of technology, which is another essential aspect of detoxing.

Some of the basic actions I've looked at throughout this book, such as increasing your intake of clean water, getting good quality sleep and chewing your food thoroughly, will have much more of a long-term detoxing effect than any flash in the pan regime. The idea of a quick fix may be appealing but engaging in lifelong healthier habits is the best way to cleanse and strengthen your body and your gut.

One element of most detoxes that I wouldn't take issue with is their emphasis on the importance of water. We need water in order to function on a basic cellular level and to support our natural detoxification processes.

quenching your thirst

Water, it seems, has acquired cult status. Carrying certain brands is seen as a statement in itself, which wouldn't be all that bad if it kept us better hydrated (except of course for the plastic bottles, but we'll come to them shortly). Adequate hydration, or the lack thereof, is something that I consistently reinforce with my clients. Many of us wonder why we have afternoon slumps, food cravings, headaches and a sluggish digestion when often it's down to simply not taking in enough water. We are made up of almost 60 per cent water and pretty much every cellular process is conducted in a watery environment, so it's no wonder that we feel tired when we don't have enough to facilitate these vital processes. Moreover, the gut is a thirsty organ and it needs regular watering to keep things moving along smoothly and regularly.

But let's be clear: you don't need to be obsessively swigging back huge gulps from plastic bottles every minute of the day. Neither should you reach the end of the day and, having realised you haven't drunk enough water, chug back litres of it. You can overhydrate too! Think 'little and often' and try to avoid drinking water with meals as this can impair optimum digestion since it dilutes the hydrochloric acid in the stomach that is crucial for breaking down our food properly. Bear in mind that you can get plenty of hydration from water-rich plant foods (and in many ways it is absorbed more efficiently from such sources), so it's not just about liquid refreshment. Foods such as watercress, watermelon, cucumber and celery contain almost 95 per cent water, although pretty much any veggie will do a decent job of hydrating you.

water quality

It's important to be discerning about the quality and source of the water you drink, so I suggest you always opt for spring water when you can. I don't want you to get dehydrated, so it is better to drink plain tap water than none at all, but it is really important to consider where your water comes from, and the purity of your tap water depends on where you live. You might consider investing in a reverse osmosis system that removes all of the impurities, including hormones, which most regular water filters won't do (I believe it's worth the investment).

When it comes to carrying water with you, forgo plastic bottles. Not only do these plastics contain possible endocrine disrupters (chemicals that can affect our hormones) but they are not so hot for the environment either, even the more eco-friendly versions. A glass bottle that you can refill is ideal, and you can get some covered with rubber – perfect when you are out and about.

Don't be fooled by some of the fancy waters out there, which do nothing more than the straight-up filtered H_2O. If you want to make your water more interesting, try adding lemon, mandolin-sliced cucumber, mint leaves, lime wedges, cinnamon sticks or even a pinch of cayenne. These can all incentivise us to drink more and they are so much better than the novelty waters that seem to be popping up everywhere.

real food

OK, so we all love a bit of a gimmick, and indulging in the latest 'superfood' powder or tonic from time to time is not a problem. But know this: eating a wide variety of foods, which are as much as possible, organic, local and seasonal, will give you the broadest nutritional value and best support for your overall health. It may not be the most innovative approach but we often overthink and overcomplicate nutrition, believing that we have to buy the most expensive ingredients when really it's about eating food in its most natural state.

These are the foods that will support you and give your body everything it needs for long-term health. Take the humble spud for example, which many people have banished from their diet. When cooked and fully cooled these beauties provide an excellent source of resistant starch that helps to feed the beneficial bacteria in the gut (check out my Punchy Potato Salad on page 62). It's the same with apples, which are a great source of fibre and antioxidants and are thought to have cardiovascular benefits (try my Stewed Cinnamon Apples on page 111). The saying 'An apple a day keeps the doctor away' has its merits so remember it when you are next tempted to overlook them in the supermarket in favour of more exotic 'super fruits'.

The obsession with the latest super foods can often be misguided. The notion that a berry that has been dried and shipped from a rainforest on the other side of the world is a better source of nutrients than freshly picked wild berries from British hedgerows is frankly silly. In fact, picking your own berries and eating them straight away ensures they are at their most nutrient-dense since they are as fresh as possible. Also, being local and seasonal, they are akin to the environment in which we are living, supported by the soil that surrounds us, so they usually yield the nutrients that we need the most. The same applies to using green powders rather than eating green veg. A simple savoy cabbage will provide you with the whole food and a more complete nutrient source. That is not to say that these powders don't have a place in the diet, and for sure they can make or break the taste of what could be just another average smoothie, but it is essential to start with *real* foods. This means cooking from scratch with ingredients in their most natural state, rather than eating foods that come in a box with heating instructions.

It's also best to think about foods individually, that is on a case by case basis, and not as food groups. For example, rather than eschewing all dairy, be discerning about the types of dairy you are consuming: opt for unpasteurised, full fat and organic as these provide us with a wealth of nutrition that you can miss out on if you ban all dairy from your diet. You will have learnt in Chapter 6 why you don't necessarily need to rule out some of these perfectly healthy foods. Indeed, focusing on the quality of the food you eat leads us nicely on to one of the other hottest debates in nutrition: are organic foods really worth the extra fuss and expense?

chemical warfare

Think about it, would you knowingly season your food with harmful chemicals? Probably not. But as grocery bills become more and more expensive, many people question the value of spending extra on organic foods. Faced with the predicament of buying one of two very similar-looking bags of spinach we may decide on the cheaper option in the belief that it surely can't make that much difference. And with plenty of scaremongering that says it's not worth the additional expense, you'd be forgiven for finding the whole debate entirely perplexing.

However, an increasing amount of research is being published showing the benefits of buying organic produce. Independent research studies by a team from Newcastle University, for example, demonstrated that the nutritional value of organic food was in fact higher than its non-organic counterpart. This included nutrients such as omega 3 fatty acids in milk and meat, thanks to the diets of the organically raised, grass-fed animals tested in the study. There were also differences in terms of vitamin and mineral content, with organic vegetables and fruit again coming out on top. The study further demonstrated that organic vegetable crops were higher in antioxidants and contained fewer pesticides.

Other research studies have demonstrated that eating organic foods equals less exposure to both antibiotics, which are predominantly ingested from non-organic animal sources, and toxic heavy metals, which are found in artificial fertilisers and non-organic soils. The same studies also linked organic foods to a reduced risk of childhood allergies, type 2 diabetes and obesity. While this research needs to be seen in a wider context, as there is no definitive answer as to whether organic is worth the extra expense, the general consensus is that you do get more nutritional bang for your buck by eating organic produce and I would certainly endorse that. So the answer to the dilemma posed by those two bags of spinach is perhaps to adopt a 'quality over quantity' approach to your food shopping.

how to prioritise when buying organic

When buying organic food make sure that it is certified as such. Look for Soil Association approval (the logo should be displayed on the packaging). This means that the food adheres to its high standards and the producer has met its environmental and animal welfare criteria. When it comes to farmers' markets, most of the producers will also proudly display this logo but don't disregard those who don't. It is definitely worth having a conversation with the stallholder, as they simply may not have gone through the certification but still follow similar practices.

Before you wince at the thought of your increasing grocery bill (farmers' markets are great for picking up deals), I'm not suggesting that everything you buy should be organic. As ever, it's about being discerning. There are some foods that really should be on your non-negotiable list, and some that you can be a bit more carefree about. The reason for this is that some produce is likely to contain more chemicals than others. It's a confusing topic but a good place to find out more is on the PAN UK and EWG (Environmental Working Group) websites (see page 270). These sites highlight the foods that are most likely to be

As well as affecting our general health, pesticides dramatically affect the health of the microbiome. This should come as no surprise, given that pesticides are designed to kill bacteria and viruses.

high in pesticides and those that pose less of a problem. These are referred to as the 'dirty dozen' and the 'clean fifteen', respectively. The lists vary between countries but tomatoes, strawberries, nectarines and cucumbers are some that rank highest globally in terms of their pesticide load. So even if it's only the top offenders that you buy organically, you've made a great start.

Another food group that is overexposed to chemicals is cereal grains. In particular they can contain high levels of the controversial ingredient glyphosate, which is commonly used in herbicides. In recent years this chemical has come under scrutiny, with the World Health Organisation deeming it a probable carcinogen. Nevertheless, it is finding its way into cereal foods, such as bread, and if we consume these chemicals regularly it can add up to quite a toxic load. As well as affecting our general health, pesticides dramatically affect the health of the microbiome. This should come as no surprise, given that pesticides are designed to kill bacteria and viruses. But studies show that a wide range of other environmental contaminants also significantly alter the composition and metabolic activity of the microbiome.

be a savvy shopper

The air miles that some of our foods rack up is bordering on insane. I mean do we really need to eat a mango in the UK in the depths of autumn, when we have apples and blackberries that are bang in season and delicious? Being more conscious of where our food has come from isn't the preserve of tree-hugging environmentalists. Yes our carbon footprint is important, but all the travelling that our food goes through to get to us also diminishes its nutritional value. Nutrients such as vitamin C, for instance, will start to deteriorate as soon as the food is harvested. So those air miles are important from the perspective of our health, as well as environmentally.

It's therefore often the case that local and seasonal food will give you more nutrients for your money. Plus it tastes a whole lot better. I don't know about you but I notice a huge difference in flavour between an apple that has come from a few miles away and one that has been flown in from the other side of the world. Hopefully, the rising trend of local artisan butchers, bakers and farmers' markets and 'growing your own' means that we will become more appreciative of the fantastic produce that can be found close to home. And why not try growing some of your own produce? You don't need a massive garden to do it. Window boxes and sprouters are a great way of tapping into your green-fingered side. Or you could try getting an allotment – that can be satisfying on so many levels.

Another way to be a savvy shopper is to limit the amount of food you waste. How often do you throw away half the contents of the fridge because you bought a ton of stuff on a whim when you were tired, stressed and hungry after a long day at work? Nobody makes good food choices in that frame of mind. Having a plan of what you are going to eat and when is the answer, as it will help you to make better choices, and save time and money. Simple things like setting up an online account for your weekly shop can be an easy way to manage this. It also saves you from being cajoled into buying supermarket BOGOFs that usually end up in the bin. Also, dedicating some time on the weekend to a bit of prep or batch cooking will pay dividends through the week.

It's also a good idea to overhaul your kitchen cupboards when you start changing your eating habits, so that you have plenty of things like dried herbs, spices and healthy oils (not bottles and jars that have been sitting in there for years). Removing the temptations will almost certainly create more clarity, determination and focus, so it's out with the old and in with the new.

Another area of concern is antibiotic-resistant bacteria, which can be present in some conventionally raised meat. Animals raised using intensive farming methods may routinely be given antibiotics to encourage more rapid growth and to prevent infection. The very real problem is that this overuse of antibiotics also leads to food-borne illnesses and infections that are increasingly difficult to treat and, as mentioned in Chapter 7, have a catastrophic effect on our gut too. However, this is not the case with grass-fed organic meat, which is why meat and dairy should really be on your non-negotiable organic list. Of course, buying meat from animals that have been treated with respect and care is also a moral consideration.

When it comes to difficult food choices, there are few topics that are more controversial than which varieties of fish we should eat. Frankly, we have dumped all manner of crap into our oceans and they are now awash with heavy metals and other such rubbish (like plastic particles) that find their way into the fish we eat. Unfortunately, there are now certain species that are so high in mercury that it is advisable to eat them only rarely. Popular choices such as swordfish and fresh tuna are thought to be the most concentrated sources of heavy metals. Not only do these metals have a major influence on the gut, they have also been associated with neurological conditions. So a good move is to opt for fish such as wild salmon (rather than farmed), as this is higher in anti-inflammatory omega 3 fatty acids and lower in antibiotics, as well as smaller fish such as sardines, herrings and anchovies, as they are lower down the marine food chain so contain less mercury. If you want to see how your preferred fish stacks up from a sustainability point of view, which is another legitimate concern, then check out the MSC (Marine Stewardship Council) website (see page 270), which explains where to look for fish that are lower in mercury.

If all this seems a little scary then remember that being aware of what you are buying and where it comes from – and any chemicals it may contain – allows you to pick your battles. Often the simple answer is to buy as much as you can that is organically farmed and from your local area. I realise that this is not always possible or realistic, of course, but doing this as often as you can supports local farmers and cuts the carbon footprint of your food too.

change is good

Making changes to your health and diet is empowering and while many of us genuinely want to embrace such changes, we naturally gravitate towards the comfortable and familiar because change is always a bit scary. However, the more we repeat something, the easier it becomes. The human body is variable, pliable in fact, and constantly changing itself, so when we start to make positive shifts we become stronger, more resilient and healthier. Our gut microbes are the best evidence of that. By re-cultivating the microbiome and helping the beneficial bacteria to flourish we can make a real, positive difference to our overall health and wellbeing. That will invariably bring about much more satisfaction than any quick-fix diet, detox or supplement.

Of course we can take inspiration from various sources, and that is what's truly great about the rising popularity of healthy eating, but each and every one of us is unique and complex, so rather than trying to fit into a mould that might be perceived as 'perfect' it's about embracing the best version of you. Find your own groove, a 'tribe' that will inspire you to move onwards and upwards, and learn new patterns of behaviour that work for you – and you'll start to experience those life-transforming changes. These don't necessarily happen overnight so be patient, give your gut the time it needs and deserves. You can be the one to make these changes literally from the next bite you take. Having a healthy gut is always multifaceted. There is no magic pill, no holier than holy lifestyle, no miraculous diet or standout form of exercise. You need a bit of all of these to give your body and your gut the fundamental support it needs. Most importantly, tune in and start to listen to your gut instinct that little bit more. Your gut will tell you when it isn't happy, and the most empowering thing you can do is to act on those signals.

That's exactly how I set out on my personal journey – probably in much the same way as you are, reading this book. Whether you simply want to improve your health or need to turn it right around, I hope I've given you some additional knowledge, a sense of empowerment and the guiding principles to start to do that, because ultimately good health begins with the true centre of our wellbeing – our magnificent and inspiring gut. Being healthy isn't about depriving yourself or spending heaps of money, as I'm sure you'll realise when you try my delicious recipes. They epitomise everything that is glorious about eating and connecting with our food and I'm sure you will make them over and over again, not just to keep your gut healthy but because you heartily enjoy eating them.

I deliberated for a long time over the title of this book but in the end decided that the message I wanted to get across was simple – *be good to your gut*. Think of your gut as a much-loved garden that you need to tend: feed it with enriching foods, weed it from time to time and water it regularly and, like any well-tended garden, it will thrive. By respecting, nourishing and giving it the support it needs you will start to experience positive changes in your health sooner than you think. Be good to your gut and it will be good to you.

spicy carrot and almond spread

Once you try this spread you will be hooked; it is super-versatile and is great for your gut! The myriad of spices – cumin, fenugreek, turmeric and cinnamon – all naturally support the health of the microbiome and provide a hit of anti-inflammatory action too. Carrots might seem like a bit of a boring veg but in fact these brightly coloured guys provide one of the best sources of beta-carotene, an important protective antioxidant, as well as supporting the immune system and the gut. Serve with Broccoli and Walnut Bread (page 226), Super Seed Bread (page 157) or Karma Krackers (page 210). This also goes great with eggs in the morning or as a nice side to some roast chicken or wild salmon. The possibilities are endless!

makes 1 small pot (serves 4–6)

3 carrots (approx. 240g)
2 tablespoons almond nut butter
25g flaked almonds
3 tablespoons extra virgin olive oil
Juice of ½ lemon
2 teaspoons ground cumin
2 teaspoons ground turmeric
1 teaspoon ground cinnamon
1 teaspoon ground fenugreek
1 teaspoon onion powder
¼ teaspoon garlic powder
Generous pinch mineral-rich salt
and black pepper

Wash the carrots and scrub with a vegetable brush; trim but don't peel them, then chop into rough chunks. Steam for 10 minutes.

Meanwhile, put all of the other ingredients into a high-speed blender. Add the steamed carrots and blend, using the tamper to push down the ingredients, or stop and scrape to get a smooth, thick consistency.

Transfer to a sealable glass or ceramic container and store in the fridge for up to 4–5 days.

nacho kale chips

Kale chips seem to be everywhere these days but they are often really expensive and nowhere near as tasty as the homemade ones. This version has a delicious nacho flavour that makes it easy to eat your greens simply by adding a generous handful as a side to your lunch. Kids love them too, so if you are trying to get them to eat more veggies these chips could be the answer. They can be cooked in a dehydrator or the oven. The value of the dehydrator method is that it retains all the nutritional benefits because it cooks at a very low temperature and thereby avoids the degrading of certain nutrients. But whichever method you use, they are easy to make, delicious to eat and gut supportive, too.

makes around 10 servings

1 large bunch kale

3 tablespoons nutritional yeast flakes

3 tablespoons almond nut butter

1 teaspoon paprika

1 teaspoon onion powder

1 teaspoon ground cumin

½ teaspoon garlic powder

Pinch mineral-rich salt

Juice of ½ lemon

Prepare the kale by cutting the leaves from the stalks and shredding them into smaller pieces. Place in a large bowl.

Blitz all the remaining ingredients in a food processor, adding a little water to thin to a smooth, creamy dressing.

Add the dressing to the leaves and massage through. If you have a dehydrator, place the leaves on the trays and set at 46°C for 8 hours. Alternatively you can bake them at the lowest setting of your oven (usually around 50°C) for 4 hours or until crisp.

Remove and leave to cool. Store in an airtight container. These will keep fresh for up to 7 days.

chicken jalapeño buns

Ariba ariba! I love these spicy burgers which have a corn twist on the buns that gives them a naturally sweeter flavour that goes perfectly with the fiery jalapeños. They are also grain free so if you are looking to find alternatives and give your gut a rest from grains for a bit then try this one. They are super-easy to make and will be a winner with all the family. Serve with mineral-rich salted sweet potato wedges and a vibrant green leafy salad.

serves 4

burgers

400g organic free range chicken mince

2 tablespoons fresh coriander

¼ teaspoon garlic powder

1 teaspoon onion powder

1 teaspoon ground cumin

2 teaspoons chopped fresh green jalapeño (or similar) chilli

Generous pinch mineral-rich salt and black pepper

buns

50g ground almonds

70 g coconut flour

50g frozen sweetcorn

3 organic free range eggs

1 tablespoon raw honey

1 teaspoon bicarbonate of soda

2 tablespoons apple cider vinegar

3 tablespoons ground flaxseed

Generous pinch mineral-rich salt and black pepper

guacamole

1 avocado

Pinch mineral-rich salt

¼ teaspoon smoked mild paprika

Preheat the oven to 180°C/Gas 4 and line a baking tray with parchment paper.

Put all the ingredients for the buns in a food processor and pulse until the mixture reaches a dough-like consistency. Divide into four and gently roll into buns. Place on the baking tray and bake for 20 minutes. Remove from the oven and allow to cool while you prepare the burgers.

Place all the burger ingredients in a large bowl and, using clean hands, mix together. Divide the mixture into four burgers and flatten. Heat a griddle or large frying pan to a medium–high heat and cook on one side for 7 minutes. Flip and cook for another 7 minutes.

While the burgers are cooking, you can make the guacamole. Remove the flesh from the avocado and mash it in a bowl, using a fork. Sprinkle with some smoked paprika and salt and work this into the mix.

Slice the buns in half, spread on a tablespoon of the guacamole, lay the burger on top and add the other half of each bun.

tip

If chicken mince is not available in your local butcher, ask them to mince some chicken breasts for you. You can also buy it online (see page 263).

celeriac and kraut rösti with poached eggs and halloumi

This is one of those anytime meals: it works brilliantly for breakfast, brunch or supper. Celeriac gives a twist to traditional rösti and packs in a decent dose of fibre for our gut microbes. Sauerkraut is a flavoursome and gut-friendly addition to the recipe. Topped with perfectly poached eggs and creamy halloumi you will come back to this time and time again. Serve with some wilted greens on the side and a decent drizzle of extra virgin olive oil.

serves 2

½ celeriac (approx. 130g)

20g sauerkraut, well drained or squeezed to remove liquid

2 organic free range eggs, beaten

2 teaspoons onion powder

2 teaspoons ground cumin

1 tablespoon coconut flour, plus 1 tablespoon for dusting

Pinch mineral-rich salt and black pepper

1 tablespoon organic unsalted butter or ghee

to serve

4 organic free range eggs

Dash apple cider vinegar

4 slices unpasteurised halloumi

Fresh herbs such as parsley or dill to garnish

Trim the celeriac then peel and grate into a large bowl. Add the sauerkraut, eggs, onion powder, cumin, coconut flour and a pinch of salt and pepper. Using your hands, mix well to combine. Divide the mixture into four and flatten into small pancakes.

Bring a pan of water to the boil, ready to poach the eggs, and add a dash of apple cider vinegar.

Heat a frying pan on a medium heat, add the butter or ghee, then add the rösti and cook for 3 minutes on each side. For the last minute or two, add the halloumi slices to the pan. Transfer the rösti and halloumi to two plates.

Poach the eggs until done to your liking. Remove and drain, then place the eggs on top of the rösti. Garnish with fresh herbs and a pinch of mineral-rich salt.

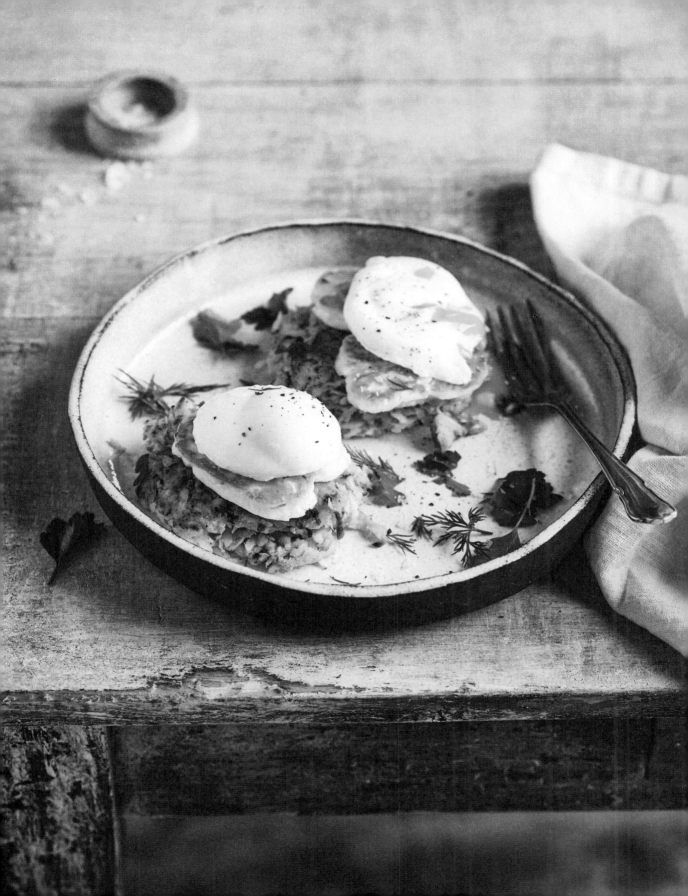

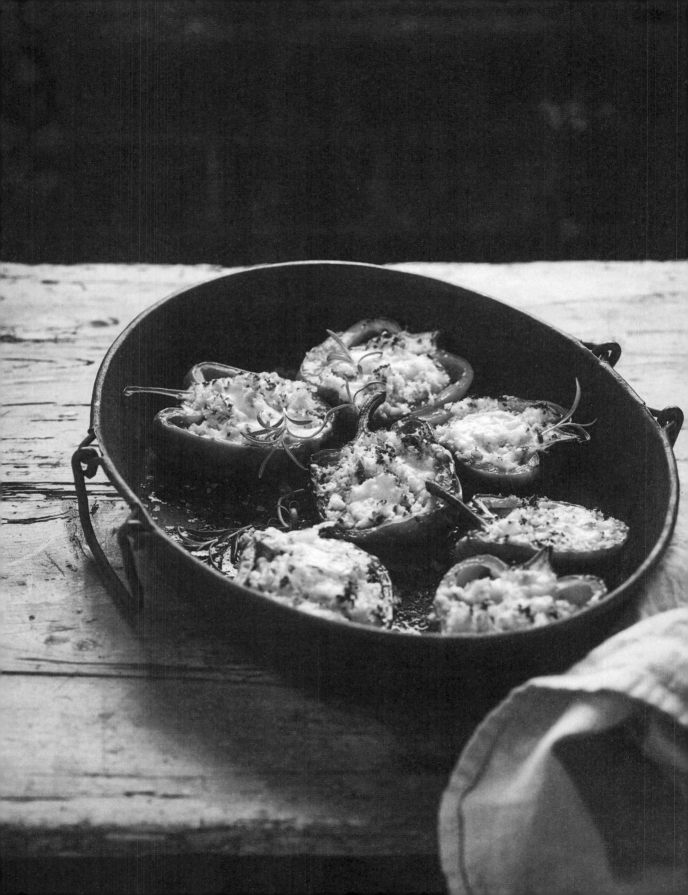

manchego, rosemary and cauli 'rice' stuffed peppers

Roasted peppers are one of those failsafe dishes that you can serve hot or enjoy cold for lunch. This recipe uses cauliflower 'rice', for a grain-free twist, and is topped with unpasteurised Manchego cheese to provide a boost for the beneficial bacteria in the gut. The fresh rosemary works as one of nature's anti-microbials and helps to manage the balance of bacteria in the gut. Best served with a green leafy salad.

serves 4 (2 peppers each)

1 medium–large cauliflower

2 spring onions, roughly chopped

2 tablespoons nutritional yeast flakes

2 teaspoons ground cumin

½ teaspoon garlic powder

2 teaspoons roughly chopped fresh rosemary

Juice of ½ lemon

Generous pinch mineral-rich salt and black pepper

4 green or red peppers

3 tablespoons melted organic unsalted butter or ghee (use coconut oil for a vegan version)

60g unpasteurised Manchego full fat cheese, thinly sliced (or 1 sliced avocado for a vegan version)

Extra virgin olive oil to drizzle

Preheat the oven to 200°C/Gas 6.

Cut the cauliflower into small florets and place in a food processor. Add the spring onions, yeast flakes, cumin, garlic powder, rosemary, lemon juice, salt and pepper. Pulse until you have a rice-like texture (about 30 seconds). You may need to stop and scrape once or twice to get an even consistency.

Cut the peppers in half and remove the seeds. Place them open side up in a deep baking dish. Divide the cauliflower mixture among the pepper halves (around 3 tablespoons per pepper). Pour the melted butter, ghee or coconut oil evenly over the peppers. Cover the dish loosely with foil and put into the oven. After 30 minutes, remove the foil and cook for a further 10 minutes.

Remove from the oven and add the cheese (or avocado), drizzle with olive oil and sprinkle with a pinch of salt.

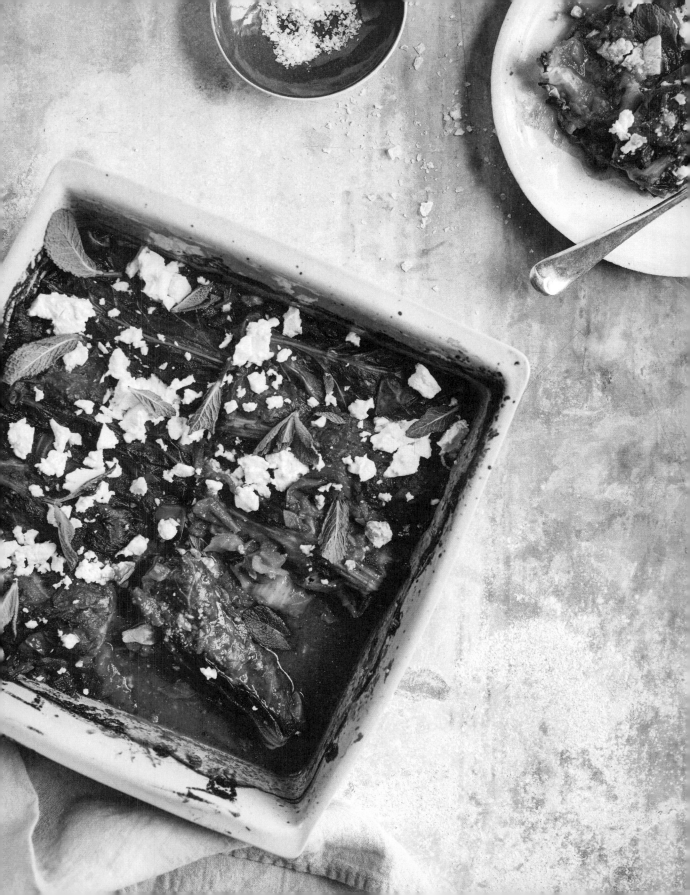

harissa lamb-stuffed cabbage rolls with feta and mint

I believe that buying organic grass-fed meat is really non-negotiable. Not just for its superior nutritional profile but also because it supports farming methods that are more sustainable and ethical. This recipe pairs sumptuous lamb with heady harissa spices and is a bit of a twist on the meat cabbage rolls we had as kids. Cabbage provides its own gut benefits: for example it is a natural source of glutamine, which helps to support the health of the gut barrier. These rolls are also mouthwateringly tasty and great for a Sunday lunch with all the family around the table. Best served with buttery green beans seasoned with a generous pinch of black pepper. And a glass of natural red wine on the side!

makes 9 rolls (serves 3–4)

1 large spring cabbage
75g unpasteurised feta
3 tablespoons fresh mint leaves, torn

lamb mixture
1 tablespoon organic unsalted butter or ghee
2 garlic cloves, peeled and crushed
½ onion, peeled and finely chopped
500g organic grass-fed lamb mince
2 teaspoons harissa spice mix
1 teaspoon ground cinnamon
1 teaspoon ground cumin
25g activated pistachio nuts, finely chopped (page 16)
1 teaspoon mineral-rich salt
¼ teaspoon black pepper

tomato sauce
1 tablespoon organic unsalted butter or ghee
1 onion, peeled and finely chopped
2 garlic cloves, peeled and crushed
400g fresh tomatoes, chopped
6 tablespoons tomato paste
400ml organic Chicken Bone Broth (page 57)
4 teaspoons smoked mild paprika
2 teaspoons dried oregano
Pinch mild chilli powder

method overleaf

harissa lamb-stuffed cabbage rolls with feta and mint method

Remove 15 cabbage leaves and trim the stalk end so it's easier to roll them. Steam for 5 minutes. Remove and leave to cool.

To make the lamb mix, heat the butter or ghee in a small pan, add the garlic and onion and cook until soft. Transfer to a small bowl and leave to cool. In a large bowl, mix the lamb mince, harissa spices, cinnamon, cumin, pistachios, salt and pepper. Add the garlic and onion mixture and use your hands to combine thoroughly. Place in the fridge.

To make the sauce, heat the butter or ghee in a saucepan and then add the onion and garlic and cook for a couple of minutes. Add the rest of the ingredients, turn the heat down to low and simmer for 10 minutes. Remove from the heat.

Preheat the oven to 180°C/Gas 4. Line a large (22 x 22cm) ceramic baking pan with 6 of the cabbage leaves. Lay out the remaining 9 cabbage leaves. Put 3 tablespoons of the lamb mixture on each leaf. Wrap the sides together and then fold the end over to make a parcel. As you make each parcel, lay it in the pan, seam side down.

Pour the tomato sauce evenly over the rolls and place in the oven for 1 hour. Remove and leave to rest for 10 minutes. To serve, crumble over the feta and the roughly torn mint.

eve's pudding

The namesake of this classic pud is one that I remember loving as a kid and my version invokes all of those comforting memories. I use honey, coconut flour and milk, which makes it creamier and also more gut friendly for those who are more sensitive or looking to reduce gluten containing flours in their diet. The honey gives a richer flavour and digestive benefits too. Serve with either whipped coconut yogurt or raw dairy cream if you really want to push the boat out and pack in some extra probiotics.

serves 8

600g dessert apples, cored and cut into chunks

50ml filtered water

2 tablespoons fresh lemon juice

1 teaspoon ground cinnamon

1 teaspoon ground allspice

sponge

100g organic unsalted butter

50g raw honey

2 organic free range eggs

50g coconut flour

200ml full fat coconut milk

1 teaspoon bicarbonate of soda

2 tablespoons fresh lemon juice

Couple drops vanilla extract

Whipped coconut yoghurt or raw dairy cream to serve

Heat the oven to 180°C/Gas 4.

Place the apples, water, lemon juice and spices in a large saucepan, bring to the boil, reduce the heat and simmer with the lid on for 8–10 minutes. Remove from the heat and set aside.

Place all of the sponge ingredients in a food processor and pulse to get a thick, pouring consistency.

Pour the apple mix into a 22 x 16cm (or equivalent) baking or ovenproof dish then pour the batter mix evenly over the top. Bake for 45–50 minutes. Test to ensure the batter is cooked using a cocktail stick – if it comes out clean, it's done.

Serve in a bowl with whipped coconut yogurt or raw dairy cream.

lemon and poppy seed pancakes

There is something absolutely heavenly about a slice of lemon and poppy seed cake with a cup of Earl Grey tea, so recreating it in digestive-boosting pancake form was a revelation! Using a base of naturally sweet coconut flour and ground almonds gives a cake-like texture with the bonus of added fibre. With zesty lemon and crunchy poppy seeds, this becomes a real treat for your taste buds and your gut. A great teatime treat or breakfast option every once in a while.

serves 1 (makes 4 pancakes)

1 tablespoon chia seeds

4 tablespoons warm filtered water

45g coconut flour, plus 2 tablespoons for dusting

¼ teaspoon bicarbonate of soda

20g ground almonds

2 teaspoons grated fresh lemon zest, plus a little extra to garnish

Juice of ½ lemon

2 tablespoons poppy seeds

3 drops of vanilla extract or seeds from 1 vanilla pod

50ml cashew milk (or use raw or unhomogenised full fat organic dairy milk, or unsweetened almond milk)

1 teaspoon coconut oil for cooking

1 generous tablespoon unsweetened coconut yogurt or sheeps' milk yogurt

Put the chia seeds and water in a bowl and leave for 5 minutes until sticky.

Sift the coconut flour and bicarbonate of soda into the bowl. Add the almonds, lemon zest and juice, the poppy seeds, vanilla and milk. Stir to combine. You should have a very thick mixture that is quite dough-like, so add more milk or coconut flour to get the right consistency if it's too wet or dry.

Take a golf-ball-sized piece of the mixture and roll it between your palms, then roll the ball in the extra 2 tablespoons of coconut flour so it won't stick to the pan and flatten to around 1cm thick. Repeat until you have made four pancakes.

In a large frying pan, heat the coconut oil and add the pancakes. Cook for 2 minutes and then turn and cook for 2 minutes on the other side. Serve on a plate, with a spoonful of coconut yogurt or sheeps' milk yogurt and a little grated lemon zest.

super hot choc

One of my all-time favourite hot chocolates is the one served at Café de Flore in Paris. And indeed the luxurious taste of that famous drink was pretty hard to match … until I made this beauty! The combination of cinnamon and star anise makes this stand out flavourwise and enhances the headline ingredient that is cacao, the purest form of chocolate. This is where it gets really interesting for our gut microbes, as they love chocolate too. That is due to the flavonols that the microbes merrily feast on, which help them to produce anti-inflammatory substances. So you can have your chocolate and eat (or in this case drink) it in moderation, knowing that it does your gut some good too. Just make sure that it's pure cacao (or cocoa) if you want to get the full benefits. This super hot choc really is a hug in a mug.

serves 1

200ml cashew milk (page 151)
2 tablespoons cacao powder
1 tablespoon maca powder
1 pitted date
Seeds from 1 vanilla pod
½ teaspoon ground cinnamon
Pinch mineral-rich salt
60ml filtered water
1 whole star anise

Put all of the ingredients, except the star anise, into a high-speed blender and pulse until thick and creamy.

Pour the liquid into a small saucepan and add the star anise. Heat gently for 4–5 minutes, stirring constantly so it doesn't burn at the bottom of the pan and you get an even temperature. Pour into a mug and sip with delight.

one-week menu planner

Planning is crucial when following the Weed, Seed and Feed programme (as it is when you're cooking from scratch as part of your everyday diet), so I've put together a one-week plan to help you get started. I always think it's best to begin on a Sunday and use that day to do some prep for the week ahead to make your life easier (see opposite for a list of recipes that can be prepared in advance). Then, each evening, you can simply make your lunch for the next day and pack your snack. It might take you a bit more time but it's going to be worth it!

day	breakfast	lunch
1	Banana Miso Honey Crumble	Crab Cakes with Cashew Dijonnaise (plus ¼ cup Sauerkraut)
2	Hazelnut, Cardamom and Cacao Granola with nut milk (or coconut yogurt)	Leftovers from Harissa Lamb-Stuffed Cabbage Rolls
3	Matcha Banana Bread with 1 tablespoon Raw Honey Kefir Cream	Beet and Fennel Burgers on Portobello Buns (plus ¼ cup Sauerkraut)
4	Pink Porridge with coconut yogurt	Sweet Potato Falafel with Parsnip 'Couscous'
5	Matcha Banana Bread with 1 tablespoon Raw Honey Kefir Cream	Nasi Goreng
6	Green Eggs and Ham	Tofu Coconut-Crumbed Dippers with Satay Sauce
7	Hazelnut, Cardamom and Cacao Granola with nut milk (or coconut yogurt)	Celeriac and Kraut Rösti with Poached Eggs and Halloumi

Note: If you are not eating lunch at home then you can use boiled eggs in place of poached or fried, so you can transport your lunch more easily.

these recipes can be made in advance for the week ahead

Tiger Nut Macaroons

Karma Krackers

Carrot and Almond Spread

Hazelnut, Cardamom and Cacao Granola

Matcha Banana Bread

1 litre of nut milk

Sauerkraut (note: ideally you'll need to do this the week before to give plenty of fermentation time)

Raw Honey Kefir Cream

dinner	snack
Harissa Lamb-Stuffed Cabbage Rolls with Feta and Mint	Tiger Nut Macaroons x 2
Cauli 'Polenta' with Shimeji and Hazelnuts	Karma Krackers x 2 with 1 tablespoon Spicy Carrot and Almond Spread
Chicken, Almond and Celery Ballotine with Wilted Chard and Creamy Caper Dressing	Tiger Nut Macaroons x 2
Miso Cod with Wasabi Broccoli	1 stewed apple with 1 tablespoon Raw Honey Kefir Cream
Wild Salmon with Carrots, Leaves and Miso Kefir Dressing	Karma Krackers x 2 with 1 tablespoon Spicy Carrot and Almond Spread
Beets and Goats' Cheese Stacks with Hemp Pesto and Butterbean Mash	1 stewed apple with 1 tablespoon Raw Honey Kefir Cream
Katsu Curry	Tiger Nut Macaroons x 2

shopping guide

kitchen cupboard

When it comes to changing your eating habits it can be really cathartic to do a kitchen cupboard overhaul and get your mind focused on what you want to achieve. Check the best before dates on stuff that's been lurking there for a while. Get rid of the less healthy temptations and stock up with inspiring and nutritionally enriching ingredients. To help you source some of the more niche ingredients in the recipes, I've put together a shopping list of items that can help you get cracking.

For most things on this list – and then some! – Planet Organic www.planetorganic.com is a brilliant one-stop shop.

Apple cider vinegar For the real deal, look for one that is cloudy, as this contains the mother culture. I like Raw Health and Bragg, both available at www.buywholefoodsonline.co.uk. Apple cider vinegar should take pride of place in your kitchen – mix it into salads, add to breads and pancakes or dilute it in a small amount of filtered water and sip as a pre-meal digestive tonic. The list of uses is endless.

Biodynamic and natural wines Isabelle Legeron MW could be called the queen of natural wine; check out her book *Natural Wine: An introduction to organic and biodynamic wines made naturally* and her website (which hosts raw wine fairs internationally) at www.rawwine.com. Other good sources are Bobby Fishel's www.gudfish.co.uk or www.buonvino.co.uk

Bone broth Make sure you always buy organic if you are not making it yourself. I love the one from Borough Broth that comes in handy frozen packets and it tastes the bomb too! www.boroughbroth.co.uk

Butter, ghee and lard My numero uno when it comes to butter is from Fen Farm Dairy www.fenfarmdairy.co.uk as it's cultured (which means it's made using a probiotic lactic culture) and made from raw (unpasteurised) milk. Otherwise you can go for Lescure cultured unsalted butter (although not organic, it does have the probiotic benefits of being cultured), available at www.ocado.com. For ghee, try Fushi Organic www.ocado.com and for pastured pork lard go to Green Pasture Farms www.greenpasturefarms.co.uk or try your local farmers' market.

Cacao Try Aduna Super-Cacao Powder, which is sourced from high-flavanol beans, available at www.planetorganic.com, and Naturya have a great organic powder as well as cacao nibs, available at www.ocado.com and health food stores nationwide. Bom Pom have both at their website www.bonpom.com

Cacao butter This is derived from cocoa beans that are pressed to remove the cocoa solids. You can buy it from health food stores nationwide or online. I like the Bon Pom one available from their website **www.bonpom.com** or on **www.amazon.co.uk**

Chestnut flour Amisa is my recommended choice here. Brilliant for baking and grain-free pancakes. Find it at **www.ocado.com**, **www.planetorganic.com** or at health food stores nationwide.

Coconut aminos This is an excellent alternative to soy sauce. Coconut Secret is a great brand that you can buy easily online at **www.planetorganic.com**, or at health food stores nationwide.

Coconut chips/desiccated coconut When buying your coconut, make sure you get the unsweetened natural versions, and not toasted.

Coconut flour A great grain-free flour. Look out for brands like Tiana that you can get at Holland & Barrett and other health food stores nationwide.

Coconut nectar blossom Biona is a great brand that you can find at health food stores nationwide.

Coconut oil For cold pressed organic coconut oil, my go-to brands are Essence of Eden, Jax Coco and Nutiva. Available at supermarkets and health food stores nationwide.

Coffee Cru Kafe is my fave organic and ethical coffee. They seek out the best beans to provide ground coffee as well as Nespresso® compatible pods **www.crukafe.com**. I also really like Roastworks, who are ethical in their sourcing and real sticklers for flavour. They call themselves 'third wave', which means viewing coffee not as a commodity but as something that should be sourced and savoured with great appreciation. I tend to agree! **www.roastworks.co.uk**

Kefir The best thing is to make your own (see page 153) using milk kefir grains (see below) and raw or organic full fat unhomogenised milk. If you are buying it, I recommend Daylesford Organic **www.daylesford.com** as they use organic full fat unhomogenised milk. Another one that I think is great is Chuckling Goat, made from goats' milk, **www.chucklinggoat.co.uk**. If you want a dairy-free version, try Rhythm Health for their coconut-based kefirs **www.rhythmhealth.co.uk**

Kefir grains Buy milk and water kefir grains to start your fermentation at **www.happykombucha.co.uk**. Once you start to cultivate them you can pass the culture on.

Kombucha If you are not fermenting your own kombucha, some great brands make it in the traditional way – my fave is Jarr Kombucha **www.jarrkombucha.com** and **www.lovekombucha.co.uk**

Lucuma and **maca powders** Natural sweeteners made from South American fruit and veg. My go-to brand for both is Naturya, which you can find in health food stores nationwide.

Matcha Lalani & Co get their organic matcha direct from family-run producers in Japan **www.lalaniandco.com**. Bloom also source their matcha organically and make some interesting blends **www.bloomtea.co.uk**

Miso paste Make sure that you buy organic unpasteurised miso paste as this means it retains all of the natural beneficial bacteria. I like Miso Tasty white or red versions **www.misotasty.com**, which are available at supermarkets nationwide.

Mushroom extract You'll find this at most health food stores. I like the Hybrid Herbs Moonrise Mushroom blend at **www.planetorganic.com** or for a more medicinal potency MycoNutri is hands down the best. Their PS-7 is a great blend of seven types of mushroom extract. Find them at **www.myconutri.com**

Nut butters Always opt for the unsweetened versions, organic if possible. Really you want just nuts and maybe a touch of salt and that's all. If you can, buy activated or sprouted versions for maximum nutritional benefits. My top brands include Profusion **www.profusionorganic.co.uk**, who have sprouted almond, cashew and hemp butter and tahini, and Damiano, who are nuts about how they source their nuts! Available at stockists nationwide.

Nut milks For the pure stuff that is just nuts, water and a bit of salt my top choice is Plenish for their cashew, almond and hazelnut milks. Find them at **www.plenishcleanse.com** or **www.ocado.com**

Nutritional yeast flakes These give a cheesy umami taste to dishes but are dairy free. Engevita is available at **www.ocado.com** and many health food stores nationwide.

Organic meat Check out your local farms and farmers' markets, but if this is not an option you can easily source online. Coombe Farm Organic is my top choice and they deliver their meats frozen **www.coombefarmorganic.co.uk**

Psyllium husks powder Kiki Health is a great brand for this. You can find it at **www.kiki-health.com** or at **www.amazon.co.uk**

Raw extracts These are pure extracts that don't contain ethanol (in contrast to most extracts) and have an exceptional flavour. Have a look at Medicine Flower Extracts, available at **www.rawliving.eu**

Raw honey Try to get honey that is as local to you as possible; look in a local health food shop or farm shop. For a choice of delicious UK-based honey and bee pollen go to Local Honey Man **www.localhoneyman.co.uk**

Raw milk There is no milk that tastes as deliciously creamy as the one from Hurdlebrook! Check out their pure raw milk and cream from Guernsey cows at **www.hurdlebrook.co.uk**. Also check out **www.johnsjerseys.co.uk** for award-winning Jersey milk and cream. And to find your local supplier head to **www.rawmilk.simkin.co.uk/index.html**

Mineral-rich salt Look for unrefined sea salt. Maldon and Halen Môn are two of my favourites. You can find them at **www.ocado.com**

Sake For premium traditionally produced sake see **www.uk.japan-gourmet.com**

Seaweed Check out Clearspring at **www.clearspring.co.uk** for their excellent selection of dried seaweed. I also love the native stuff from the Cornish Seaweed Company **www.cornishseaweed.co.uk**

Seeds I particularly like Organic Traditions; they also produce sprouted flaxseed and chia, which are generally better absorbed by the body. They also sell hemp hearts (shelled hemp seeds). Find them at **www.planetorganic.com** or at health food stores.

Spices and **herbs** are a mainstay of any kitchen pantry. Get yours well stocked up and use them for inspiration and to raise any dish to another level of flavour. Look at Steenbergs **www.steenbergs.co.uk** for a great selection of organic herbs, spices and blends or head to The Spice Shop **www. thespiceshop.co.uk**, renowned for its incredible spices.

Sprouted grains When it comes to grains, then sprouted or fermented is best for your gut. Check out Rude Health for their sprouted oats and flours at **www.rudehealth.com** or Planet Organic for their own-brand sprouted oats, quinoa, amaranth and buckwheat at **www.planetorganic.com**

Tea Making a pot of tea can be a relaxing and restorative ritual in itself. There is no one that specialises in craft single-batch teas direct from the growers like Lalani & Co. Behind every tea is a story and some incredible tastes. Check them out at **www.lalaniandco.com**. I also like Joe's Tea Co for some awesome flavours **www.joesteacompany.com**

Tempeh Impulse Foods source 100 per cent organic and GMO-free soya beans that are fermented in the traditional way to create the tastiest tempeh. Find them at health food stores nationwide or at **www.impulsefoods.co.uk**

Tiger nuts and powder These sweet little tubers are amazing for the gut. The Tiger Nut Company provides them in various forms, including powder and flour **www.thetigernutcompany.co.uk**

Tofu Make sure you get 100 per cent organic and GMO-free tofu. Clean Bean stick to the most natural and traditional processes and you can really taste it in their tofu **www.cleanbean.co.uk**. Another good brand is The Tofoo Co **www.tofoo.co.uk**

Unhomogenised full fat milk Duchy Organic is available at **www.ocado.com** and Waitrose stores. Daylesford Organic is available at **www.daylesford.com** and **www.ocado.com**

Unpasteurised cheese For an exceptional range of ewes' cheese head to **www.homewoodcheeses.co.uk** or **www.thecourtyarddairy.co.uk** who can deliver direct to your door.

kitchen kit

Investing in a few bits of kit can transform your recipe repertoire and make it fun and easy to prepare gut-friendly food. For accuracy you will also need digital kitchen scales, which you can buy almost anywhere. Here are some of my top choices.

Blender Hands down the best high-speed blender in the biz is a Vitamix. It does *everything* and is well worth the investment. Have a look at the smaller versions if you are making meals for just one or two people **www.vitamix.co.uk**

Ceramic knives Keep your veggies as fresh as possible by using ceramic knives that don't cause immediate oxidisation like other knives. Check out Kyocera for the best quality ones **www.kyoceraknives.co.uk**

Dehydrator To activate your nuts and seeds by soaking and then drying, a dehydrator can be very handy. You can use a low oven, but the dehydrator works at a very low temperature and retains all the nutritional benefits. Have a look at the Excalibur models at **www.ukjuicers.com**

Food processor My favourite is made by Magimix; spending a bit more on a good quality processor means it will last longer **www.magimix.uk.com**

Kitchen utensils Good quality peelers, mashers, spatulas and graters will help you achieve top-notch results. Malle w.Trousseau is often my go-to, available at **www.mallewtrousseau.com** or find their products at **www.madeindesign.co.uk**

Pots and pans Spend more and buy yourself a set of pans that will last a lifetime and are not coated with chemical nasties. I love Crane Cookware **www.cranecookware.com** and Le Creuset **www.lecreuset.co.uk** or Green Pan, whose pans are made from non-stick ceramic **www.greenpan.co.uk**

Spiraliser Have fun with your veggies by putting them through a spiraliser. The Hemsley + Hemsley one is great, or try Lurch. You can get both easily on Amazon and at selected retailers.

Sprouters These are cheap and cheerful and can be used to grow lots of different sprouts, which can add a nutritional kick to salads and veggies; they can even be added to smoothies. Check out **www.ukjuicers.com**

water and filtration systems

Bottles Ditch your plastic bottle and invest in a snazzy rubber-cased glass ones to carry around **www.mybkr.com**

Filtration The guys at the Pure H2O Company know more than a thing or two about water. They specialise in reverse osmosis systems; if you want more info head to their website at **www.pureh2o.co.uk**

supplements

I believe that gut health begins with food first and foremost, which means following the principles outlined in the Weed, Seed and Feed programme (page 46). However, supplements used in the right way and for the right reasons can help support this process. With this in mind, here are some of my recommended choices. Note: always consult your doctor or registered practitioner if you are taking any medications or believe you might have contra-indications.

Anti-microbials Supplements that could be useful as part of the Weed, Seed and Feed programme to target bacterial overgrowth include Tigon Wild Oregano Oil and Biotics Research Garlic Plus. Find these at **www.revital.co.uk** or **www.naturaldispensary.co.uk**

Enzyme Science Digestive Enzymes These can help support reserves that may be depleted, which can contribute to symptoms such as bloating or indigestion **www.enzyscience.com**

Nutri Advanced Glutagenics L-glutamine powder that helps to support the health of the lining of the gut **www.nutriadvanced.co.uk**

Symprove A liquid probiotic; the website includes research to highlight the efficacy of their formula **www.symprove.com**

Vital Nutrients Betaine HCL Pepsin Gentian Root Extract If you suspect your stomach acid levels are 'not keeping up with the Joneses' then taking a betaine hydrochloride (HCL) supplement can help boost them naturally. Try the baking soda test first (page 73) to see if this may be of benefit **www.vitalnutrients.net**

Vitamin D Wild Nutrition food-grown vitamin D is a good option if your levels are on the low side. Available at **www.wildnutrition.com**

natural beauty products

Food isn't the only thing that can affect the microbiome. The products we put on our skin and the cleaning products we use in our home also have an impact. The best place to source natural beauty products that focus on high performance and results is **www.contentbeautywellbeing.com**. You will find innovative brands such as DeMamiel, May Lindstrom, MV organic skincare and Ilia Beauty, to name a few.

dress your table

I've talked in the book about the importance of *how* we eat and connect with our food; dressing your table is a big part of that. When you have spent time preparing and cooking, your food deserves to be showcased appropriately. That means getting some attractive dishes, cutlery and linens. Here are some of my fave brands but check out markets and antique stores too for some real bargains.

The Cloth Shop Vintage glassware and *the* place to pick up some of the most beautiful linens **www.theclothshop.net**

Cutipol Delightful cutlery that has you savouring every last bite **www.cutipol.pt**

Mud Australia Delightful porcelain in some of the most exquisite colours. These will make your dishes even more stand-out **www.mudaustralia.com**

Summerill & Bishop Tableware and tablecloths – this place is a mecca for elegant dining **www.summerillandbishop.com**

resources

lab testing and other analysis

British Gut Project is an open source crowdfunded project headed by Professor Tim Spector, which provides data on the diversity of your gut microbiome. It does not offer interpretation though, so you will need to seek the advice of a registered practitioner **www.britishgut.org**

Genova Diagnostics run all manner of functional tests that include comprehensive stool analysis, hormone profiles, cortisol saliva testing and food sensitivity and allergy panels. These need to be run with your registered nutritional practitioner – see below for details on how to find one locally **www.gdx.net**

Map My Gut – gut microbiome 'mapping' analysis and interpretation available through a registered practitioner **www.mapmygut.com**

registered nutritional practitioners

BANT (British Association for Applied Nutrition & Nutritional Therapy) – use the website to find a registered nutritional therapist in your area **www.bant.org.uk**

BDA (British Dietetic Association) – use the website to find a registered dietician in your area **www.bda.uk.com**

CNHC (Complementary & Natural Healthcare Council) – a national voluntary regulator for complementary healthcare practitioners where you can find registered therapists local to you **www.cnhcregister.org.uk**

IFM (Institute for Functional Medicine) – the institute that coined the phrase 'functional medicine', which addresses the underlying causes of disease using a system-based approach and lab testing for personalised treatments. You can find a certified practitioner at the website **www.functionalmedicine.org**

environmental and organic organisations

EWG (Environmental Working Group) – US-based non-profit organisation with consumer guides on many health and environmental issues including pesticides and additives **www.ewg.org**

Farmers' markets – check out FARMA (National Farmers' Retail & Markets Association) to find your local markets and farm shops **www.farma.org.uk**

FDA (US Food & Drug Administration) provides a comprehensive list on the mercury concentration in fish **www.fda.gov**

MSC (Marine Stewardship Council) – details on the sustainability and traceability of your fish of choice **www.msc.org**

PAN UK (Pesticide Action Network) for info on pesticides and how you can support more environmentally conscious initiatives **www.pan-uk.org**

The Soil Association is the UK's leading charity for healthy, sustainable and ethical farming practice and land use. It is also the UK's largest organic certification body – always look for the Soil Association stamp when buying organic **www.soilassociation.org**

further reading

Here are some of my stand-out books on gut health, microbes, mushrooms, misconceptions about food and our connection with it.

Eat Right, Nick Barnard (Kyle Books, 2016)

10% Human, Alanna Collen (William Collins, 2015)

Gut, Giulia Enders (Scribe, 2015)

The Diet Myth: The Real Science Behind What We Eat, Tim Spector (Weidenfeld & Nicolson, 2015)

The Big Fat Surprise, Nina Teicholz (Scribe, 2015)

How to Eat, Thich Nhat Hanh (Parallax Press, 2014)

First Bite, Bee Wilson (Fourth Estate, 2016)

I Contain Multitudes, Ed Yong (Ecco, 2016)

Medicinal Mushrooms: A Clinical Guide, Martin Powell (Mycology Press, 2014)

The Art of Fermentation, Sandor Katz (Chelsea Green Publishing Co, 2012)

The Ethical Carnivore, Louise Gray (Bloomsbury Natural History, 2016)

sources

If you want to read about the studies and research related to the book, please visit my website for a full listing **www.evekalinik.com**

glossary

This A–Z glossary will help you familiarise yourself with some of the technical terms used throughout the book.

a

Adrenaline A stress hormone, also known as epinephrine, produced in the adrenal glands in response to a signal from the brain. It sends messages around the body to prepare for fight or flight, for example by increasing the heart rate and blood flow to the muscles. See also cortisol.

Amino acids Used in every cell of the body, these compounds form the building blocks of protein, which is necessary for growth, repair and regeneration, and they are vital for the production of enzymes, hormones and neurotransmitters. They also play a crucial role in the storage and transportation of nutrients and metabolic processes. In the body there are twenty amino acids (known as standard amino acids), of which nine are 'essential' for humans, meaning that they cannot be made by the body and need to come from our food.

Amylase An enzyme that is produced in saliva glands and in the pancreas in order to break down carbohydrates into simple sugars.

Antibody/Antigen An antigen is a protein expressed by a bacteria or virus (usually on its cell surface) that is recognised by the immune system as 'foreign'; the immune system then responds by producing an antibody (aka immunoglobulin). Some antibodies create an extreme response, such as the anaphylactic reaction of immediate swelling of the tongue or throat after eating an allergen; other antibodies are working constantly to counteract pathogens in the gut.

Antioxidants Molecules found in a variety of foods, particularly vegetables, fruit, nuts and seeds, or produced in the body, that help to protect cells against damage by oxidation.

b

B cells Part of the immune system, these are white blood cells that make antibodies in response to antigens and develop 'memory' for these antigens for when the immune system comes into contact with them in the future.

Bile A yellow/green liquid that is produced by the liver to help digest and absorb fats (and stored in the gall bladder).

Bolus The small ball of food chewed in the mouth that then makes its way to the stomach.

Butyrate A short-chain fatty acid made by bacteria in the gut that is the major source of energy for colon cells, supports the intestinal barrier and has anti-inflammatory benefits. Also found in higher amounts in foods sources such as unpasteurised cheese, ghee and organic or cultured butter.

Cholecystokinin (CCK) The hormone that is released in response to fat from chyme as it enters the small intestine. It stimulates the release of digestive enzymes from the pancreas and of bile from the gall bladder.

Chyme The mush of food in the stomach that makes its way to the small intestine.

Cortisol A stress hormone produced in the adrenal glands in response to a signal from the brain. It sends messages around the body to prepare for fight or flight, for example by increasing blood sugar and negatively affecting digestive processes. See also adrenaline.

d

Dysbiosis An imbalance between beneficial and potentially pathogenic bacteria that can have a negative impact on the gut and overall health.

e

Enzyme A type of protein needed for chemical reactions throughout the body. Digestive enzymes are used to break down the nutrients from our food.

Fibre The non-digestible part of carbohydrates that makes its way to the colon for our microbes to 'eat' and produce beneficial substances and nutrients.

Free radicals Molecules that can damage cells by oxidation and cause inflammation in the body. Antioxidants can limit this damage.

GALT (Gut-Associated Lymphoid Tissue) Lymphoid tissue of the gastrointestinal mucosa that lines and protects the gut. Responsible for localised immunity to pathogens such as bacteria and parasites.

Ghrelin The 'hunger hormone' that sends a signal to the brain saying it's time to eat.

Glucagon This hormone plays a part in blood sugar regulation. It works with the liver to stimulate the conversion from glycogen to glucose, which is released to raise blood sugar levels when they drop too low. It also works in a process called gluconeogenesis, which is the production of new glucose from non-carbohydrate precursors such as amino acids.

Glucose A simple sugar that serves as the primary fuel for metabolic processes and energy in the body.

Glycogen Stored and readily available glucose that can be released to regulate blood sugar levels and provide energy when needed.

h

Homeostasis A state of balance and equilibrium in the body. Various systems work to maintain a constant internal environment that ensures the body operates optimally, including regulation of body temperature and volume of water in the body.

Hormones Chemical messengers produced by glands and specialised cells throughout the body. They communicate between organs and tissues on a wide range of activities, including digestion, respiration, sleep and reproduction.

i

Insulin The hormone that is released when we eat and our blood sugar levels rise. In response, insulin signals for glucose, our primary fuel, to be shuttled into cells, ready for use. Insulin also controls excess stores of glucose and either stores it as glycogen in the liver or deposits it in fat tissue. It also communicates to the hypothalamus in the brain to suppress appetite so we know when to stop eating.

Intestinal epithelium The layer of cells that lines the small and large intestines and separates the gut (and the substances we have ingested) from the rest of the body.

Intestinal villi and **microvilli** Finger-like projections that line the small intestine; they assist with absorbing nutrients into the bloodstream.

l

Leptin A hormone produced by adipose (fat) tissues that tells the brain when we are full and suppresses appetite.

Lipase The digestive enzyme that is responsible for breaking down fats.

Lipid The scientific term for fats and oils.

Lipopolysaccharides (LPS) Toxic substances found in the cell membranes of certain types of pathogenic bacteria that can create inflammatory responses in the body.

m

Macrophages Part of the immune system, these are white blood cells that act like Pac-Men, gobbling up cellular debris and other foreign matter.

Microbiome or **microbiota** The entire bacterial population on, or in, the body. The majority of this is found in the gut.

Microorganism or **microbe** A tiny organism that may live on, in or around us and can only be seen through a microscope. They can be divided into six types: bacteria, archaea, protozoa, algae, fungi and viruses. Some are beneficial, some superfluous and some harmful. The human gut houses trillions of microbes.

Minerals and trace elements Essential nutrients found in various foods and needed by the body for a wide variety of functions. They include calcium, chromium, copper, iodine, iron, magnesium, potassium, selenium, sodium and zinc.

Mucosa A mucus-secreting membrane that lines part of the body such as the gut or respiratory tract. The gut mucosa has a number of roles: it helps with protection of the gut, absorption of nutrients and secretion of substances needed for digestion.

n

Neurotransmitter Meaning 'nerve messengers', these are chemicals that communicate between neurons (nerve cells) and other cells (in nerves, muscles and glands). As such, neurotransmitters manage our thought processes and moods, as well as involuntary processes such as blood circulation and digestion.

o

Omega 3 A type of oil known as an essential fatty acid: 'essential' means it cannot be produced by the body and needs to come from our food. Omega 3 is crucial for brain health and for anti-inflammatory action throughout the body.

p

Pathogens Organisms such as parasites, certain types of bacteria, fungi and yeasts that can disrupt the equilibrium of the gut and may contribute to digestive symptoms and associated conditions, particularly when they reach high numbers.

Pepsin The enzyme in the stomach that helps to break down protein.

Peptide YY (PYY) An appetite-suppressing hormone that the small intestine releases in response to eating. It slows down the passage of food to increase nutrient absorption.

Phytochemicals or **phytonutrients** Beneficial compounds found in plants (such as fruit, vegetables, nuts, seeds and herbs) and plant-based foods (such as tea, coffee, chocolate and spices).

Polyphenols In terms of nutrition, these are specific types of phytonutrients. Flavonoids are a type of polyphenol found in coffee and chocolate.

Prebiotic Foods containing certain types of fibre that 'feed' the beneficial microbes in the gut.

Probiotics Beneficial bacteria or yeasts that have a positive role in the body. They are found naturally in the gut and in fermented foods. They can also be taken in supplementary form.

Serotonin A neurotransmitter, often described as the 'happy hormone' because it influences mood and contributes to feelings of wellbeing. More than 90 per cent of our serotonin is produced in the gut.

Short-chain fatty acids (SCFAs) Beneficial substances, such as butyrate, produced by bacteria in the large intestine from insoluble fibre. SCFAs provide energy for the colon's cells and support the immune system, among other roles.

T helper cells White blood cells that support the activity of other cells in the immune system to regulate an appropriate immune response. They release substances called cytokines that activate B cells to produce antibodies and instruct other T cells to kill abnormal cells.

T-regs cells Immune system cells that communicate with the microbiome and coordinate other cells to help manage healthy immune responses. They have a modulating role rather than an activating role.

Vitamins A range of nutrients that are vital for the healthy maintenance of cells throughout the body. Some vitamins come from our food; others are made in the body.

Yeast Microorganisms classed as part of the fungus family. Naturally occurring or 'wild' yeasts have been used for millennia to make bread and beer. Other species of yeasts, such as *Candida albicans*, can act as pathogens and potentially damage the gut.

index

acknowledgements

Firstly I'd like to thank my family and friends – without them none of this would have been possible. Thanks to my little bro for being you and always having my back. To Sarah, who is one of the most positive souls I have ever met and continues to inspire me; your strength is such a virtue. To Nat – who, during that life-changing time in Mexico, convinced me to pursue my dream in nutrition – thank you for always pushing me onwards and upwards. To my other Nat and her darling Tats; without your consistent support, artistic input and impeccable taste I don't know where I would be. To Niamh, for telling me what's what – your straight-up honesty and fearless opinion always set me straight. And to my boys: Alan, Dale, Kevin, Gito, Vincent, Keith and James – you are a fabulous lot. I'd also like to thank David, who didn't call me crazy when I decided to take a different career path, and was there to help me manage the tremendous task of studying and working (you are also the best ice cream taster ever!). And to the magical Sonia; I do not know how I would have kept it together without you.

Thanks to my outstanding team: to Georgie, for being you and for being my biggest fan (and now one of my closest friends); to Jules, my right-hand girl; and to Aaron, I truly value your talent, hard work and kindness. You are the best.

To those who have championed me from the start and helped get me on the right path, thank you – without you guys I wouldn't be here writing this book. Stephen, you put your trust in me right at the beginning of my career and have believed in me ever since, I have so much respect and gratitude towards you. To Emine, words can't describe how much I have come to love you for so many reasons; thank you for giving me all of the opportunities you have so gracefully sent my way; I look forward to so many more exciting moments together. And to Kara, I hope your formidable business acumen and sharp-witted thinking have caught on, you are brilliant. To Ruth, who so generously gave me that first editorial platform at matchesfashion and continues to endorse my work. And to Calgary, who has consistently supported me right from the start of this journey. You are all so inspiring.

Thanks to my pals in the industry who continue to do such incredible work. Sometimes the path isn't always easy but I truly admire all your tenacity and creativity – Nick, Ian, Imelda, Jas & Mel, Ross and Barry & Carol. Keep on keeping on.

Thanks also to the incredible team that pulled this book together. My publisher Zoe and editor Jillian, you understood the vision and throughout this process your enthusiasm and patience have made this book better than I ever imagined possible. To my agent Juliet, who I knew was the girl for me the moment we met and also got me, too. Thanks to the wonderfully talented photographer Nassima: I never thought my recipes (and me, come to that) could look this good, and to the gorgeous Rosie for styling them so beautifully. And to the personal styling team – Jenelle, Christel, Suman and the girls at matchesfashion.com – for making me look pretty decent.

To all my clients – you are the reason why I wrote this book and every one of your stories reminds me of why I wanted to do this job in the first place.

And lastly, this book is dedicated
to my mum and dad. You have
never once doubted me and I feel
truly lucky to have you both in
my life. Love you to bits.